LIVE LONGER, LIVE BETTER

LIVE LONGER, LIVE BETTER

LESSONS FOR LONGEVITY FROM THE WORLD'S HEALTHIEST ZONES

MELISSA PETITTO, R.D.

chartwell
books

Quarto

This edition published in 2023 by Chartwell Books,
an imprint of The Quarto Group
142 West 36th Street, 4th Floor
New York, NY 10018 USA
T (212) 779-4972 F (212) 779-6058
www.Quarto.com

10 9 8 7 6 5 4 3 2 1

Chartwell titles are also available at discount for retail, wholesale,
promotional, and bulk purchase. For details, contact the Special Sales
Manager by email at specialsales@quarto.com or by mail at The Quarto
Group, Attn: Special Sales Manager, 100 Cummings Center Suite 265D,
Beverly, MA 01915, USA.

ISBN: 978-0-7858-4200-2

Library of Congress Control Number: 2022947483

Publisher: Wendy Friedman
Senior Managing Editor: Meredith Mennitt
Senior Design Manager: Michael Caputo
Editor: Jennifer Kushnier
Designer: Kate Sinclair

Photo credits: **Shutterstock**/Tom Jastram: 6; Kit Leong: 50.
Alamy/Marina Saprunova: 67; Alberto Maisto: 153. All other stock photos
and design elements (except pages 33, 38, 46, 63, 85, 93, 98, 108, 112,
and 145) ©Shutterstock.

Printed in China

INTRODUCTION

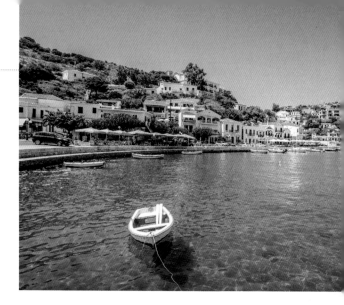

The fountain of youth—also known as eternal youth or even the mythical fountain—was a term originally coined by early explorers Ponce de Leon, Panfilo de Narvaez, Hernando de Soto, and many others searching for a fabled spring whose very waters were thought to rejuvenate one's youth and health. That search for eternal youth didn't die with the explorers.

Today, we are subjected to the all-encompassing world of the multimillion-dollar beauty industry. An industry that includes, but is not limited to, anti-aging, cosmetics, cosmetic surgery, hair care, weight loss, fragrances, personal care, acne care, and so much more. An industry that promises us a magic pill that delivers immediate weight loss, a salve that gets rid of acne overnight, a serum that reverses fine lines and wrinkles in just two weeks, a hair oil that reverses hair loss. We have all bought into the assurances at one time or another—I know I have!

But what if we are looking at the aging process all wrong? What if, instead of reversing the signs of aging, we fully embrace all the knowledge and wisdom gained from it and age with grace? What if we focused on aging for longevity and living a pain-free, disease-free existence into our later years? We have beautiful examples from around the world to show us that this very phenomenon is not only possible but is actually quite simple to achieve.

Sardinia, Italy was first studied by Gianni Pes and Michel Poulain while doing demographic work for the journal *Experimental Gerontology*. They identified Sardinia's Nuoro province as a region with the highest percentage of male centenarians, or people who live to be 100 years old. Not only are these people living to be 100 years old and greater, but they're living without dementia, disease, and other health problems.

Upon learning about this region and the healthy lives its inhabitants lead, I became hooked, selfishly needing to know more. My reason: My dad is getting older, something we all have to deal with and learn how to handle as the child becomes the adult caring for aging parents. My dad's health has taken some curveballs lately, ones that make his life a little more difficult for my mom to manage. I wanted to figure out ways to help them on this journey, allowing them to have the best possible later years of life. Though it's a self-serving reason, who among us does not want that for our parents, our grandparents, and truly for ourselves and our children?

After Sardinia was studied, more regions were found to have some of the same characteristics of long-living, healthy people: Loma Linda, California, where the Seventh-day Adventist Church population leads the United States in the longest life expectancy; Nicoya, Costa Rica, where life hasn't changed much in decades and yet lives are longer and healthier than in any other country on earth; Ikaria, Greece, where napping seems

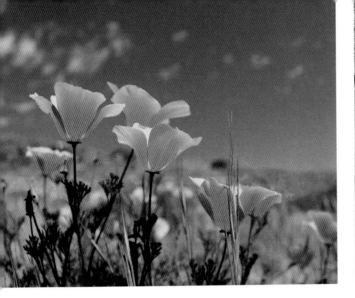

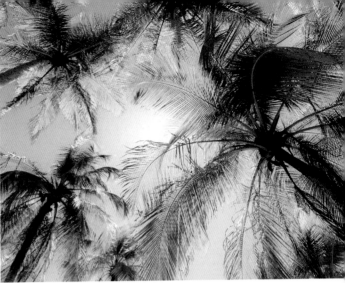

to be a secret of these long-living people; and Okinawa, Japan, where it's believed that a strong social network and community extends lives.

What do these people know that we don't? How did they find the so-called "fountain of youth" without the beauty industry's multimillion-dollar answers? I wondered the same thing. In this book, I present my discoveries. In it, you will learn the simple—and sometimes incredibly basic—ways that the people of these diverse regions stay mentally sharp, physically active, and disease free into their later years.

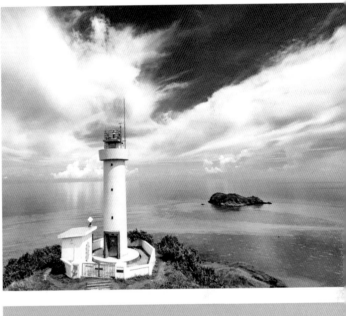

Since this is a cookbook, I would be remiss if I didn't mention that most of my findings tie back to food. Each of these communities have such beautiful connections to the earth and the food they prepare from it. They naturally eat seasonally, locally, and (for the most part) organically. I will include some of their unique ingredients in each chapter. Some might be a little tricky to find, but I will always give direction as to where to look for them, as well as simple swaps that might be a little easier to locate. But do try to find the unique ingredients if you can—they are extremely nutritious, and they just might be the secret to each community's longevity.

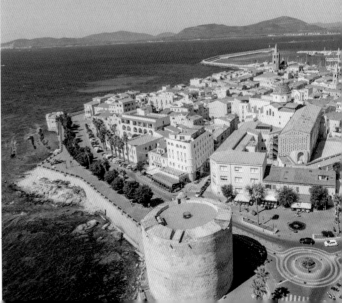

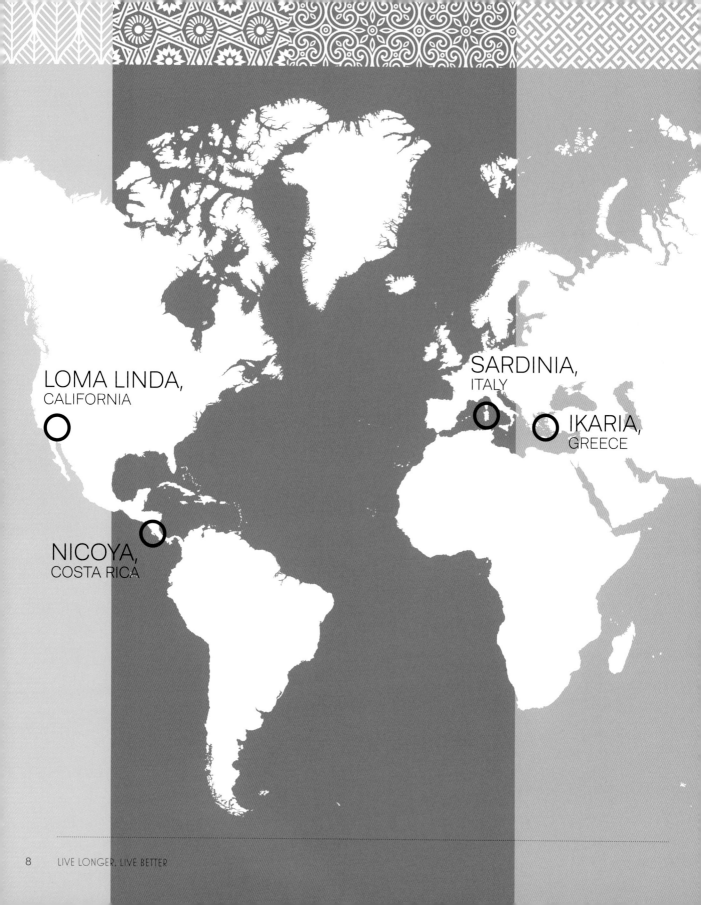

LOMA LINDA,
CALIFORNIA

SARDINIA,
ITALY

IKARIA,
GREECE

NICOYA,
COSTA RICA

CHAPTER 1

THE 10 TENETS OF LONGEVITY

These five locations from all around the world have something in common: the people of these places live longer and healthier lives than in any other place on earth. You would think there was a secret that they all knew, a food they all consumed, an herb they ingested every day, but the true reason behind their health and longevity is multifaceted. Upon careful reflection and study of these different peoples, I've found that they share ten main lifestyle habits or beliefs that help them maintain their youth and vigor.

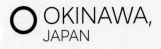 OKINAWA, JAPAN

(ONE) MOVE SIMPLY

The people of these regions believe that movement is a natural part of one's life. While most people in our society think 30 to 90 minutes of high-impact exercise is the definition of movement in life, these areas of the world have redefined what movement and its link to longevity and health means. They include movement as a daily ritual, whether that's walking to a friend's home or gardening. Movement not only decreases the risk of certain ailments related to inactivity, but it also contributes to better mental health. Studies have shown that movement decreases anxiety and depression by increasing serotonin levels. Movement can also keep the mind sharp as we age. The key here is that it is a natural part of daily life and that it's dynamic, not static. It is living on a steep slope and walking up or down to get to the store; it's dancing late into the night in celebration; it is riding your bicycle to the neighbors or community gathering; and it is gardening for your family and friends.

AILMENTS RELATED TO INACTIVITY

- Obesity
- Colon, breast, and uterine cancers
- Depression
- Anxiety
- Heart disease
- Type 2 diabetes
- High blood pressure
- Osteoporosis
- High cholesterol and lipid disorders
- Stroke
- Metabolic syndrome

10 SIMPLE WAYS TO INCLUDE MOVEMENT IN YOUR DAILY ROUTINE

1. Make time; 30 minutes is all you need
2. Park in the back of a parking lot and walk
3. Take the stairs instead of the elevator or escalator
4. Do some housework
5. Garden or mow the lawn
6. Ride your bike or take a simple walk
7. Walk the dog a few extra blocks
8. Ask for support from your friends and get them involved
9. Try new activities with your family
10. Have an accountability buddy

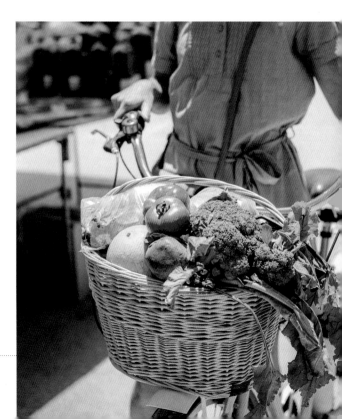

In Okinawa, they call it *ikigai*; in Nicoya, it's *plan de vida*. Both phrases translate to "reason to live." The belief in one's self, the knowledge of why you are here and what you bring to the world around you, gives individuals a reason, a purpose, each and every day of life. The slow way of life that inhabits these five places gives great meaning to "a reason to live." Each resident has a job, a purpose for their day, whether it be to provide food for their family, to watch the grandkids, to herd the sheep, or to make the herbal tonics for their family or neighbors. Life has meaning in the everyday tasks that others may find menial, but that truly make life worth living. Many studies have shown that having social bonds is an essential source of meaning in life, which builds community engagement, which then creates a society that thrives.

HOW TO INCLUDE PURPOSE IN YOUR DAILY LIFE

- Start a gratitude journal
- Write down what and who you wake up for daily
- Create a vision board of the life you envision
- Have a growth mindset
- Give back
- Explore passions
- Join a community endeavor
- Spend time with people who inspire you

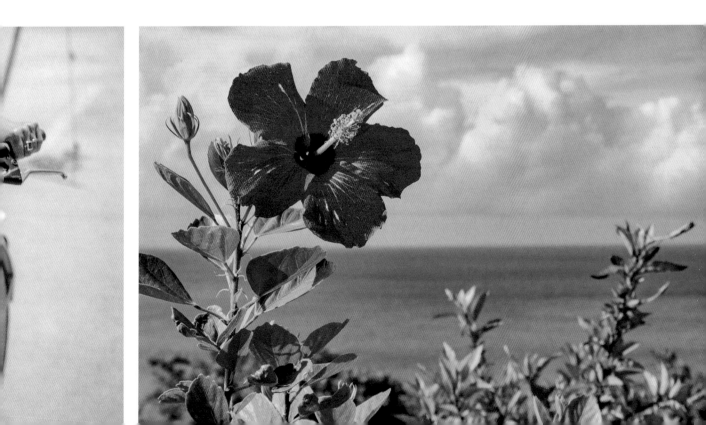

(THREE) SLOW DOWN

Inflammation, a term we've become all too familiar with in today's world, is the root cause of a lot of age-related diseases—and stress is a leading cause of chronic inflammation. Though stress is a part of everyone's lives, people who live the longest and healthiest include stress relief as a natural part of their daily ritual. For example, in Okinawa, the daily routine includes the remembrance of ancestors; in Loma Linda, the Adventists pray daily; in Ikaria, naps are a part of the regular schedule; in Nicoya, an afternoon siesta comes after the hard work of the morning routine; and in Sardinia, happy hour brings a time to unwind. In our modern world, most people view stress as something that is inescapable, but to the people residing in these areas of the planet, life is about living and loving life, not stressing out about the pressures of high-tech work, long commutes, and overpacked schedules. The emphasis on life in Loma Linda, Okinawa, Sardinia, Nicoya, and Ikaria is not defined by financial productivity but rather love, community, and family.

10 NATURAL WAYS TO DE-STRESS

1. Be physically active
2. Meditate
3. Unplug from electronic devices
4. Laugh
5. Get a massage
6. Take a bath
7. Read a good book
8. Cook as a family
9. Write in a gratitude journal
10. Listen to music

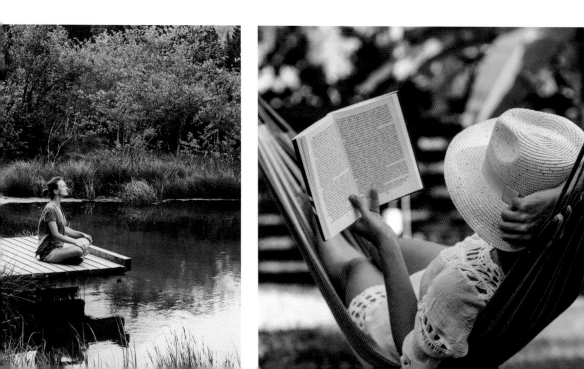

PRACTICE MINDFULNESS

Mindfulness is not a new concept; in fact, its roots reach back to religious and secular traditions, from Hinduism and Buddhism to yoga and, most recently, nonreligious meditation. This practice that has been around for thousands of years is one that teaches the beauty of a pause. In yoga it is called *kumbhaka*; translated from Sanskrit, it simply means suspension or retention of breath. The power of the pause teaches us to stop at the top or bottom of a breath, to take a breath during a moment to experience something in its entirety, and to live in the present.

Okinawans have a phrase, *hara hachi bu*. This is a 2500-year-old Confucian mantra that reminds the diner to eat only until 80 percent full. The concept allows the diner to slow down, eat mindfully, and allow their body to feel the food consumed, letting it nourish the body wholly. There is a modern notion of eating and feeding our bodies that is so disconnected from this act of eating mindfully. (When was the last time you wolfed down fast food in your car or grabbed a granola bar on your way out the door?) To enjoy our food that was grown with our own hands, to dine with friends who are our family, and to lengthen the dining experience, turning it into a ritual not a chore...this is what it means to eat mindfully.

These simple ways to add mindfulness to your day are not just about eating, but about living a more centered, fulfilled life. When you start noticing the beauty in the little moments, those little moments accumulate to become the memories that make up our lives. Studies about mindfulness show that when it is included as a part of everyday life, our lives are less stressful, our moods are brighter, our anxiety is decreased, and our health is greatly and positively impacted.

10 SIMPLE WAYS TO ADD MINDFULNESS TO YOUR DAY

1. Turn off all electronics during meals
2. Practice gratitude
3. Do a body scan and check in with how you are feeling
4. Stop and ask your heart how it is feeling
5. Stop and check in with your five senses
6. Take a deep breath or three
7. Put down your fork in between each bite; savor each one
8. Listen fully and with intention
9. Walk barefoot on the grass, beach, or soil
10. Stop and look around; notice where you can find the beauty in the everyday

(FIVE) EAT PLANTS (MOST OF THE TIME)

Most people in these regions consume small amounts of meat. The main component in each of these places is fresh fruits and vegetables, with the foundation being lentils and beans—fava, soy, and black. Eating plant-based has so many health benefits, ranging from improvement of the gut biome and better absorption of nutrients from your food, to improving your immune system and reducing inflammation. Eating real, whole foods, not processed ones, is paramount to living a long and healthy life. Let's take a closer look at these benefits.

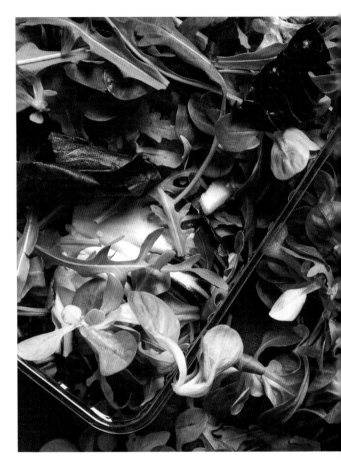

1. IMPROVING THE GUT BIOME Studies show that eating a high-fiber diet of plant-based foods contributes to a wide range of prebiotics that nourish the beneficial bacteria of the gut. Prebiotics act as fertilizers that stimulate the growth of these healthy gut bacteria. There's even been evidence linking a healthy gut biome to better health—both physically and mentally.

2. BETTER ABSORPTION OF NUTRIENTS While eating a plant-based diet can improve your gut health, it also allows the nutrients to be better absorbed. High-fiber foods such as beans, legumes, and vegetables help to sustain optimal blood sugar and cholesterol and increase the absorption of minerals such as iron and calcium. Plants also have essential nutrients that you cannot get from other foods. These vitamins, minerals, phytonutrients, and antioxidants help keep your cells healthy and your body in balance so that your immune system can function at its best.

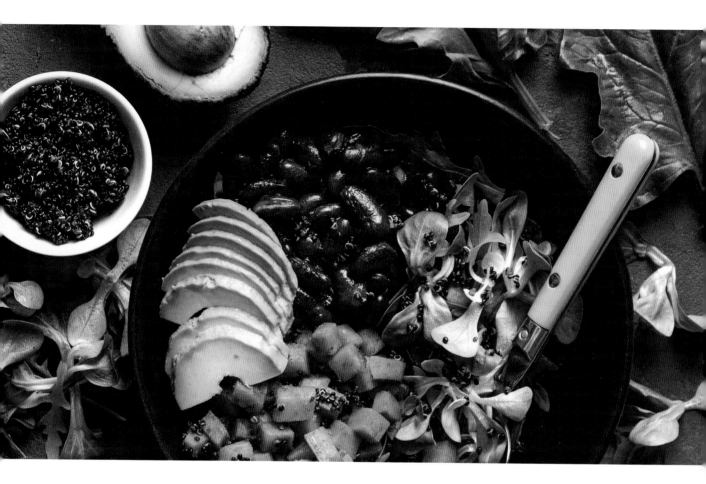

3. IMPROVING YOUR IMMUNE SYSTEM Your immune system is crucial for lowering your risk of cancer by identifying and attacking mutations in cells before they can progress to disease. Plants give your body the ammunition (in the form of antioxidants, phytochemicals, vitamins, and minerals) it needs to help ward off infection. A plant–based diet also helps to strengthen the immune system, which protects you against microorganisms and germs.

4. REDUCING INFLAMMATION The essential nutrients in plants help to reduce inflammation in the body. The same phytochemicals and antioxidants that boost your immune system are the same ones that counterbalance the toxins from processed foods, bacteria, viruses, and pollution. Extended exposure to these toxins can damage your body's cells and tissues and is linked to cancer and other inflammatory diseases such as rheumatoid arthritis, osteoarthritis, fibromyalgia, and lupus.

SIX

ENJOY WINE (IN MODERATION)

In most of these five cultures (the Adventists excluded), wine, often homemade, is enjoyed nightly over dinner with friends and family. Wine includes antioxidants and polyphenols that have been shown to reduce the risk of heart disease and certain cancers, and slow the progression of neurological disorders like Alzheimer's and Parkinson's disease. (But don't worry, the benefits of wine are strong whether it's homemade or not.)

In moderation, wine has been shown to dilate blood vessels and increase blood flow, which lowers the risk of blood clots and damage to the heart muscle. Wine also appears to raise levels of HDL, or good cholesterol, and helps stop LDL, or bad cholesterol, from damaging the lining of arteries. The polyphenols in wine also seem to limit the oxidation of LDLs, making them less efficient at damaging those artery linings, which in turn lowers the risk for cardiovascular disease, heart disease, and stroke. Red wine is often seen as the most beneficial alcohol because of resveratrol, a compound found in the skin of grapes. Because red wine is fermented with the grape skins longer than white wine, red wine contains more resveratrol.

WHERE TO FIND RESVERATROL IF YOU DON'T DRINK ALCOHOL

1. Simply eat grapes or drink grape juice. The amount of resveratrol is not the same, but you can still seep up some of the benefits by eating and drinking grapes/grape juice.

2. Eat peanut butter, blueberries, and cranberries. While the amount of resveratrol is not the same in these foods, there is some—and that's better than nothing!

3. Eat dark chocolate. It's a good source of resveratrol!

4. Take supplements. Research is lacking on the body's ability to absorb resveratrol from supplements, but they are out there and do seem to provide some benefits. (Talk to your healthcare provider before adding any supplements to your diet.)

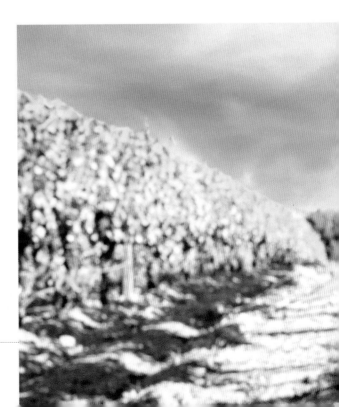

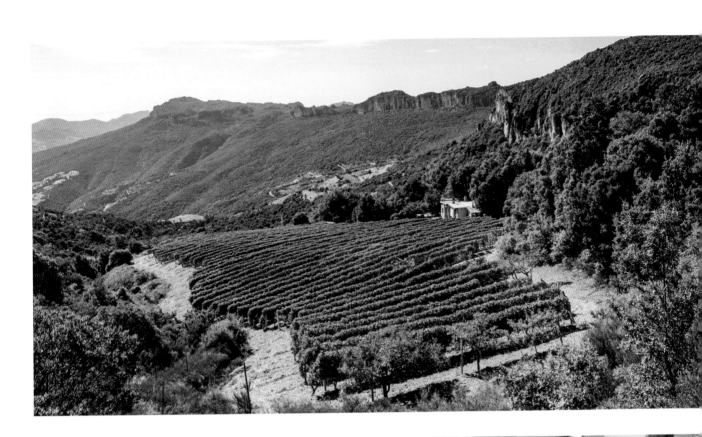

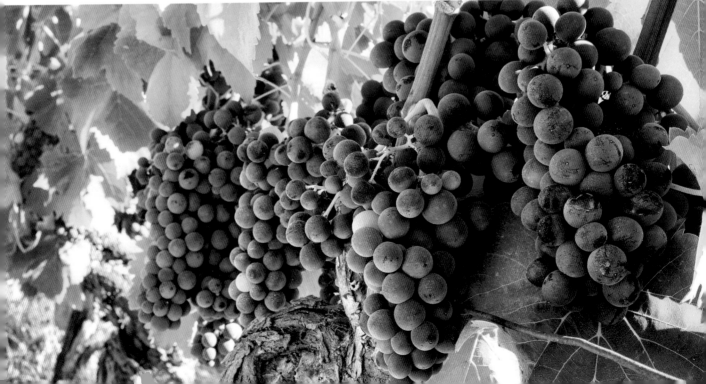

(SEVEN) FIND YOUR PEOPLE

Your family, or your chosen "found family," is one of the most important factors in your health journey. In Okinawa, the term *moai* is used to describe a group of five friends who choose to commit to one another for life, and in Ikaria, communities are very close and choose to socialize frequently. Chosen groups that maintain positive habits, like supporting one another throughout their lives, have been shown to extend life and help promote health. Research has shown that with that kind of support, one's life is elongated *just by knowing* that love and support are there if needed. In fact, one study showed that more than 80 percent of centenarians communicate with a friend or family member daily, and that this one factor has increased their survival rate by 50 percent!

I know from personal experience that both my chosen family and the family I was born into are pillars of strength that make life that much richer. I know that when times are hard and when times are incredible, I turn to the people who support me no matter what, who believe in me always, and who are my greatest cheerleaders. It isn't always an easy task to find friends as we age, but having an open mind and heart are a good starting point.

10 WAYS TO MEET LIKE-MINDED PEOPLE

1. Join a group activity (book club, community theater, ski club, running club, quilting circle, tennis or pickleball group)
2. Volunteer in your community
3. Join an amateur sports league
4. Try a new class at the gym or at a local community college
5. Join a Zumba or dance class
6. Join the PTA
7. Join a cultural or religious group
8. Join a wine club
9. Join a Meetup
10. Host a neighborhood get together

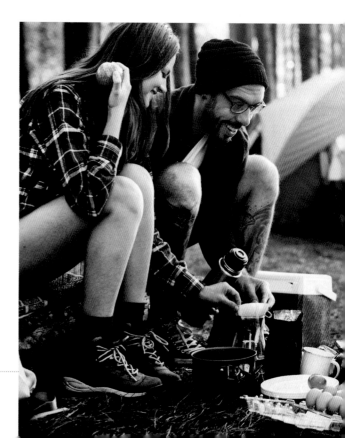

EIGHT

FAMILY FIRST

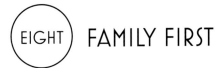

Family always comes first in these five regions around the world. This shows up in many forms: aging parents and grandparents living in or near other family members and being a part of daily life; committed, healthy, and positive relationships; and caring for their children by investing time, love, and energy. There have been many studies that show that having grandparents as a part of grandkids' lives is mutually beneficial: grandparents feel appreciated, and they get to share their lives with the next generation, teaching their grandchildren to respect and keep traditions; the grandchildren learn these traditions, stories, and recipes from their elders.

Grandparents can help alleviate household stress by being available to watch the grandchildren, doing light household tasks, or baking family favorites. In turn, grandchildren help maintain and even boost their grandparents' cognitive performance. If you think of the dozens of questions little kids ask—and all the times they want to play with everything from crayons and puzzles to dress-up and other games of imagination—all of this is stimulating to an older person's brain. Grandchildren also help increase grandparents' immune systems by exposing them to all of the immune-building germs that kids come into contact with. Finally, grandchildren help bring a purpose to the grandparents' lives, which in turn lowers their risk of depression. Even if you live far away from your extended family, technology makes it easier than ever to maintain those relationships; scheduling the time to do this (and perhaps teaching the grandparent how) is worth the effort.

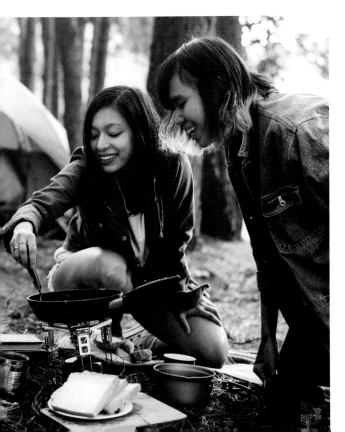

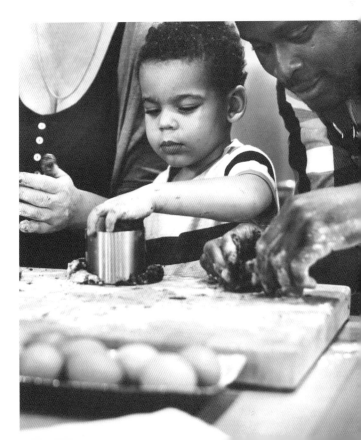

(NINE) FIND YOUR FAITH

Another piece of the longevity puzzle in these areas of the world is the belief in something bigger than one's self. Belonging to a faith–based community builds strong social relationships, which can add years to one's life. Whether you are in an organized religion or spirituality is more your thing, the positive impact on your mental health is the same. Both teach a person to tolerate stress by generating peace and purpose. Both believe in community and offer a sense of belonging in a social environment. Both offer ritual, structure, and predictability, which help with coping when there is a difficult life situation to navigate. Both offer compassion, forgiveness, and gratitude. And both provide an opportunity to look within and recognize or come to terms with the meaning of life and decipher where we fit in.

I have never been one that fits into the structure of organized religion, often feeling like an outsider in the synagogue where I was raised. As a Southerner, being raised Jewish was hard enough, but coming from a mixed religious family was even harder. My dad is Catholic, and my mom is Jewish, and I grew up in Alabama. Faith was tangible in Alabama, something that was everywhere I looked. Judaism is something I have always felt is a part of myself culturally, but spiritually, I was a child who asked questions and those questions led me to finding a deep and beautiful spirituality practice. At 21, I found yoga, which held my heart and my soul more than anything ever had before. I wish for everyone to find that peace, that acceptance, that part of you that trusts in the unknown. Explore, have an open mind, and find what makes sense for you.

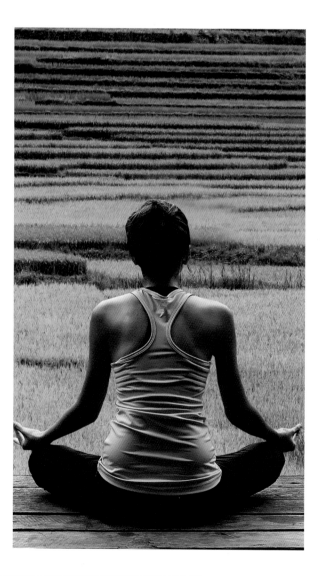

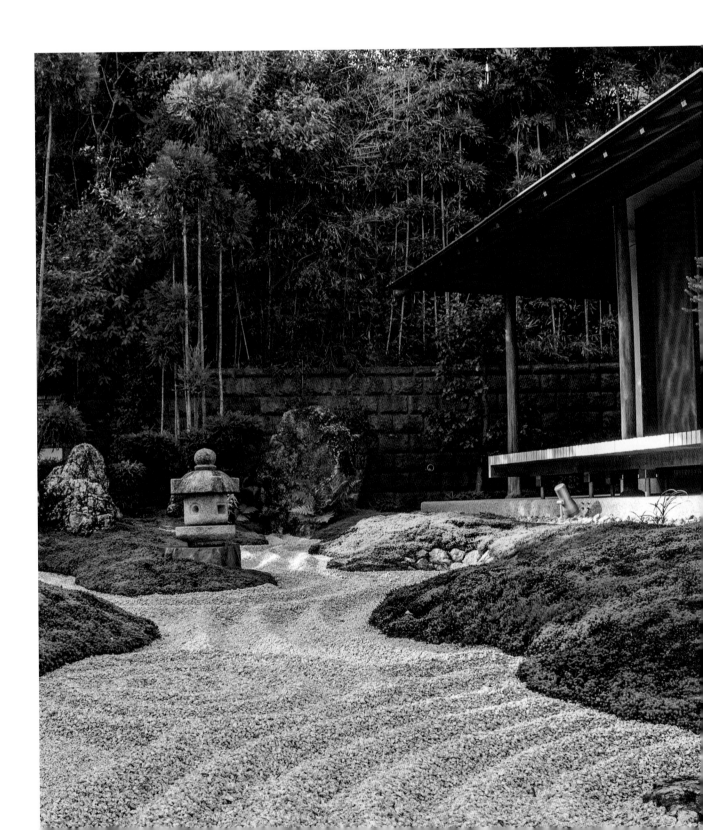

FOOD EQUALS FAMILY

The last similarity between these peoples, the final tenet of how to live longer, better, is food. Food is enjoyed with friends, food is enjoyed with family, food is enjoyed with community. Food is to be shared, to be honored, to be eaten with reverence and taken in as enjoyment as well as nourishment. Among all these different cultures, food is what brings people together over love, laughter, and the belief that what we put into our bodies should be locally sourced, grown with our own hands, and seasonally appropriate so that it's loaded with vitamins, minerals, and nutrients.

WAYS TO SHARE FOOD

- Serve or cook for a local food bank
- Start a dinner club
- Visit a farmers' market
- Meet the farmers that grow your food
- Go apple, pumpkin, blueberry, or strawberry picking
- Have a weekly or monthly potluck dinner with friends
- Prepare a family recipe as a family
- Bring a neighbor dinner or some baked goods

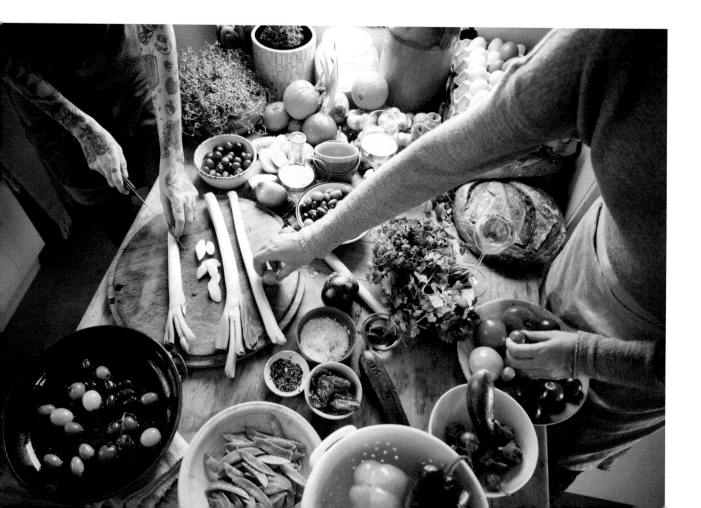

A RECIPE FOR LIFE

After reading the principles that the people of Okinawa, Sardinia, Ikaria, Nicoya, and Loma Linda have in common, the main takeaway is that the secret to a long and healthy life is not just about what we eat. Food is a major part of our lives. Food brings joy, food means family, food provides nourishment, food is pleasure—but combined with the other nine principles these areas of the world share, this equals a recipe for a life that is full of love, purpose, health, and longevity.

That said, there are a few similarities in nutritional and eating habits that I noticed while researching these communities:

EAT WHOLE FOODS Each of these communities eats whole foods and very little processed foods. When beginning this journey, try to eat as many natural and whole foods as possible.

DRINK MOSTLY WATER When I was little, I had an aversion to water; in fact, my family nicknamed me "the camel" because I never drank fluids. No one can say that about me now! I always have a huge travel water with me. It might take some getting used to, but staying hydrated is one of the easiest ways to nourish your body and skin, lubricate your joints, regulate your body temperature, and deliver nutrients to your cells.

LIMIT SUGAR This is possibly the one habit I feel strongest about. Increased sugar intake has been directly linked to inflammation, elevated blood pressure, fatty liver disease, diabetes, weight gain, and so much more. I'm not saying these communities omit sweeteners altogether; while do they enjoy more natural sweeteners such as fruit and honey, sweets tend to make fewer appearances. If you begin eating whole, less-processed foods overall, it will become easier to limit your daily sugar intake.

LOVE YOUR LEGUMES Members of each of these communities regularly eat beans and other legumes. This habit has so many obvious health benefits, including increased fiber content and loads of vitamins and minerals. But there's a benefit that might not be as obvious: when you are eating beans, less meat is needed (or eaten) to feel full. Plus, beans and legumes are incredibly versatile and delicious!

GRAZE ON NUTS I love this habit and am guilty of carrying my favorite nuts with me everywhere. I pull them out and snack on them whenever I am feeling a little tired and in need of an energy boost. (My toddler and her friends tell me I have the best snacks!) As I'll share in the coming pages, nuts are an amazing source of antioxidants, vitamin E, magnesium, and omega-3 fatty acids. Start setting yourself up for success by packing some nuts so you always have the ultimate brain food on hand.

This doesn't sound so hard, does it? So let's take a journey around the world and look at some of the delicious dishes that are typical of each region, placing emphasis on the plant-rich ones. Eating plant based is a passion of mine, and the people of these diverse locations thrive by putting plants first in their lives. I'll discuss the main ingredients used in each area, defining the health benefits of each. These ingredients are a huge part of the traditional make up of each place but are by no means the only ones that are utilized. For each area, I'll also give tips on how to include small portions of the meats and seafood that are sometimes included. Let's dive in.

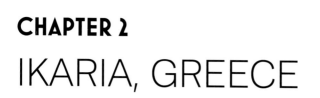

CHAPTER 2
IKARIA, GREECE

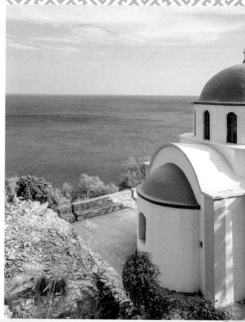

Ikaria, Greece, is an island in the Aegean Sea, off the coast of Turkey. It is a land of Mediterranean climate, of organic farming, and of robust community. The population is about 8,500 permanent inhabitants and, according to research by the Faculty of Medicine at the University of Athens, almost the entire population is free from chronic diseases and dementia—and sexually active well into their late 80s. Traditional ways of life are agriculture, livestock farming, and, to a lesser degree, fishing. Ikaria's landscape is rugged and lush, dotted with rivers, waterfalls, gorges, enormous boulders, cool turquoise waters, and breathtaking sunsets.

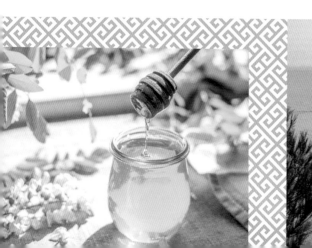

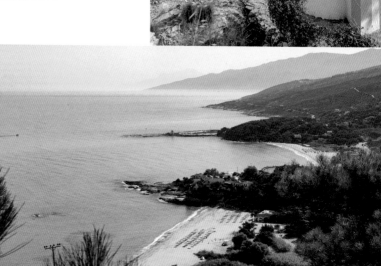

A Day in the Life

Tourists often find Ikaria a peculiar place, a place where the traditional timing of shops opening and closing does not apply. The people of Ikaria tend to let their nights be the focus of their day-to-day lives. In the village of Christos Rachon, shops open around midnight and stay open until dawn. Ikaria may have its own clock, but the hospitality to visitors and those in need is unparalleled. Travel between villages is difficult, but residents make it a little easier by opening their homes, hearts, and kitchens to care for road weary travelers.

The island of Ikaria is also known for its tradition of *panagiria*, or festivals. During the months of May and October, the island hosts between two and four festivals per week. In other parts of Greece, most of these *panagiria* are held to celebrate a religious holiday, but in Ikaria they are held mainly to just celebrate—celebrate life and community. These all-night feasts of boiled or grilled goat, fresh vegetable salads, and sixteen-proof red wine are followed by dancing. Lots and lots of dancing. The festivals tend to raise money that then goes back to the village, whether for the church or the infrastructure.

Most days start a little late in Ikaria with, I am told, a spoonful of Ikarian honey. The honey is used as a medicinal preventative, a perfect start to the day. The roads are not very well paved on Ikaria, so most people tend to stay within their villages where they not only grow their own food, but also work the land, and then cook the very food that was procured that day. It's a beautiful and simple way of life, but not an easy one.

The traditional Ikarian diet is one of simplicity, moderation, variation, and seasonality, with the spare use of meat. The diet has always been both a foraged and a homegrown one. The day normally starts with a late breakfast consisting of goat's milk yogurt or cheese, fruits, herbal tea or coffee, whole-grain bread, and local honey. This simple meal seems just that, but the health benefits of these few items are astounding. The herbal tea is a rich and vital tradition to Ikarians. It is an important part of the local culture, as both food and folk medicine. Seasonal herbs such as marjoram, sage, mint, chamomile, rosemary, and dandelion are brewed into restorative hot and cold teas that provide antioxidants and other properties.

A large lunch after working in the gardens is a necessity. Salads are made of beans, legumes, and potatoes, fresh daily caught fish, picked-that-day vegetables, and tons of olive oil. Homemade wine is also enjoyed at this meal, as is love, laughter, and community. An afternoon nap tends to follow the big meal, a time to rest before going back out to work the land. This practice makes for a stress-free work routine.

Dinner is often a simple fare of bread, olives, foraged or homegrown vegetables, and more wine. This tends to be a time where neighbors visit and catch up on the day. Around midnight, bedtime follows a fruitful, tiring, and love-filled day.

The Food of Ikaria

Ikaria is known as the Greek island where people forget to die, and their diet is a huge part of that longevity! The Ikarian diet is mainly based on what grows in and around the island. Very similar to the Mediterranean diet, the emphasis is on plant-based ingredients with fish, other seafood, and meats making a minimal appearance. The cuisine is distinguished by its moderation, simplicity, and contrast. Ikarians eat seasonally, utilizing wild greens and other wild vegetables they forage for on the hillsides, tons of olive oil, honey, wild lupin beans and other legumes, and fresh herbs. There is no commercial farming in Ikaria, so everything grown is organic. Here are a few of their mainstays.

WILD GREENS *Horta* is the term Ikarians used to define the edible greens and herbs that are gathered and consumed in the island's mountains, fields, and gardens. These greens are wild, dark, and rich in vitamins and iron, magnesium, potassium, calcium, and carotenoids.

POTATOES These tubers are not often considered a healthy vegetable, when in fact they are full of antioxidants, which prevent disease; they're a good source of fiber, potassium, and magnesium, which help maintain healthy bodily functions. They're also low in cholesterol and sodium. The resistant starch fiber in the potato, which has benefits of both soluble and insoluble fiber, has been shown to help prevent heart disease by keeping cholesterol and blood sugar levels in check.

LENTILS The lentil is one of the oldest and most common superfoods. These potassium-, folate-, and iron-rich legumes have been shown to lower blood pressure, protect the heart, support the formation of red blood cells, help fight off fatigue, and, for those who are pregnant, aid in the development of the fetus.

GARLIC This bulbous plant in the allium family is truly a miraculous medicinal addition to savory food. Garlic naturally helps boost the body's immune system, helps reduce high blood pressure and cholesterol levels, is a cancer preventative and antibiotic, may help prevent Alzheimer's disease and dementia, and has been shown to enhance athletic performance. Rich in vitamin C, vitamin B_6, and manganese, it also contains trace amounts of various other nutrients. Eating garlic regularly has also been shown to help detox the body of heavy metals.

FRESH HERBS Fresh herbs (particularly basil, dill, mint, and oregano) are used in abundance in Ikarian cooking. Basil is high in antioxidants and contains anti-inflammatory and immune-supportive properties, supports the nervous and digestive systems, lungs, liver, and brain. Dill aids in digestion, helps fight infections, and supports healthy cholesterol levels; it helps relieve coughs, supports the kidneys, and boosts immunity. Mint is an appetite stimulant and is great for digestion and calming the intestinal tract. Oregano is a powerful antibacterial, antifungal, and antiviral; it is also a strong anti-inflammatory.

LEEKS Leeks are another member of the allium family. The leek is considered a superfood for its flavonoid richness, particularly one called kaempferol. Kaempferol is an antioxidant that has anti-inflammatory, antidiabetic, and anticancer properties. Leeks have been shown to lower the risk of prostate, stomach, colon, and esophageal cancers because of their ability to repair damaged DNA. Leeks are also rich in vitamin K, which has been shown to lower the risk of osteoporosis. This little vegetable also contains lutein and zeaxanthin, which help to protect the eyes from cataracts and macular degeneration. Besides vitamin K, leeks also are a good source of manganese, copper, folate, iron, vitamin C, and vitamin B_6.

OLIVE OIL Olive oil is a cornerstone of the Ikarian diet, and its benefits are incredibly powerful. Olive oil is proven to reduce inflammation and may help prevent strokes, heart disease, cancer, diabetes, and Alzheimer's disease. It is also a natural antibacterial agent. One study out of Ikaria found that olive oil consumption is more powerful than Viagra.

HONEY Raw honey has been used for generations as a preventive medicine. The honey used in Ikaria is pure, unfiltered, and raw; it is super rich in antioxidants, including flavonoids, phenolic acids, carotenoid derivatives, and amino acids. The nectar used by bees includes that of blossoming sage, pine, lavender, and wild oregano, and is thought to create an especially healthy honey that is rich with vitamins, minerals, and antioxidants. Honey is a natural antibiotic and antibacterial wound healer. It contains many anticancer properties, is a natural cough remedy, and has been shown to boost energy. Honey reduces inflammation, and the high vitamin C content has been shown to speed the growth of healthy tissue in the body.

FIGS Both the fruit and the leaves of figs are packed with nutrients. They have been shown to promote healthy digestion, aid with constipation, and are a natural prebiotic, which helps to feed the good gut bacteria. Figs are particularly rich in copper and vitamin B_6. Copper is a vital mineral that aids in metabolism and energy production, as well as the formation of blood cells, connective tissues, and neurotransmitters. Vitamin B_6 is essential to helping the body break down dietary protein and create new proteins. It also plays a key role in brain health.

NUTS Almonds, walnuts, and chestnuts are some of the most commonly eaten nuts on Ikaria. Nuts are an amazing source of antioxidants, vitamin E, and magnesium. They help lower the bad cholesterol, control blood sugar levels, and help reduce inflammation. They are also rich in omega-3 fatty acids, which are an incredible anti-inflammatory aid that helps with brain health.

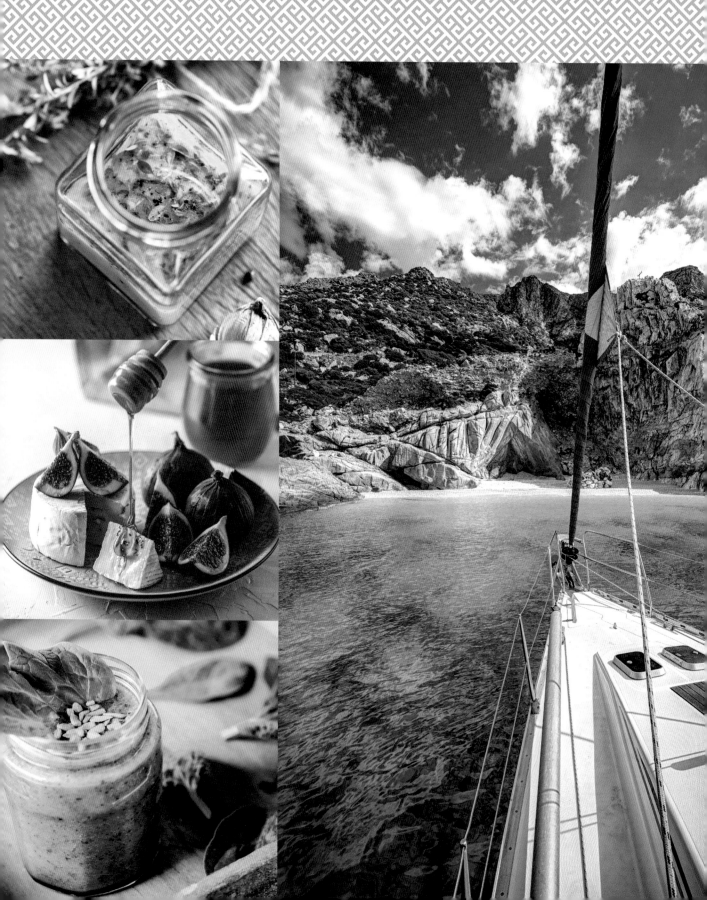

The Recipes of Ikaria

GREEK YOGURT WITH HONEY, FRESH FRUIT, AND TOASTED ALMONDS

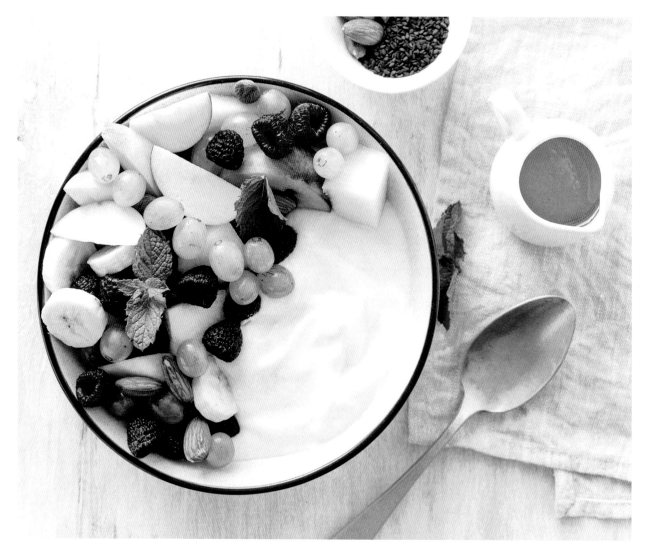

A traditional, no-fuss Ikarian breakfast, this dish is so versatile. It changes year round, depending on the fruits of the season. Get creative and showcase what nature provides! The base of great quality Greek yogurt and raw local honey pair perfectly with all seasonal fruits. You can even play with spices if you want; try sprinkling with cinnamon in the fall and winter for a naturally blood warming breakfast.

Serves 4

¼ cup (22 g) sliced almonds

2 cups (254 g) plain Greek yogurt, plant-based or regular

2 cups (300 g) mixed fresh fruit, such as raspberries, melon balls, grapes

2 tablespoons (43 g) raw local honey

1. To toast the almonds, warm a small sauté pan over medium-low heat. Add the almonds and stir, tossing gently for 5 to 7 minutes, or until the almonds are lightly browned and fragrant. Watch them carefully to avoid burning. Remove from heat and transfer to a small bowl to cool slightly.

2. Divide the yogurt between 4 bowls. Top with the mixed fruit and toasted almonds. Drizzle with the honey.

Honey is used for both savory and sweet dishes on Ikaria. You could easily leave the greens off this dish and serve it with some yogurt for a healthy and beautiful dessert. Fresh figs are in season during the summer but are abundant for just a short period of time. I grew up with a fig tree in my Alabama backyard, and in August we feasted on figs every which way we could. This recipe, where the fig shines in all its glory, reminds me of those childhood days.

Serves 4

8 ripe figs

¼ cup (86 g) raw local honey, divided

½ cup (60 g) roasted, salted, shelled pistachios, chopped

1 tablespoon (15 ml) good quality balsamic vinegar

2 tablespoons (30 ml) Greek extra-virgin olive oil

4 cups (2 oz [57 g]) mixed baby greens

½ teaspoon Maldon or other flaked sea salt

¼ teaspoon freshly ground black pepper

1. Preheat the oven to 375°F (190°C, or gas mark 5). Line a baking sheet with parchment paper.

2. To prepare the figs, cut in half through the stem and lay cut side up on the prepared baking sheet. Drizzle with 2 tablespoons (43 g) of the honey.

3. Transfer to the oven and bake for 15 to 20 minutes, or until soft and bubbly. Allow to cool for 5 to 10 minutes.

4. While the figs are cooling, prepare the pistachios. In a small sauté pan over medium-low heat, add the remaining 2 tablespoons (43 g) honey and pistachios. Allow to come to a simmer. Remove from heat and stir in the balsamic vinegar and olive oil.

5. To serve, arrange the figs on a large platter, mound the baby greens on top, drizzle with the pistachio dressing, and finish with the flaked sea salt and black pepper. Serve immediately.

WARM FIGS WITH HONEY AND PISTACHIO DRIZZLE

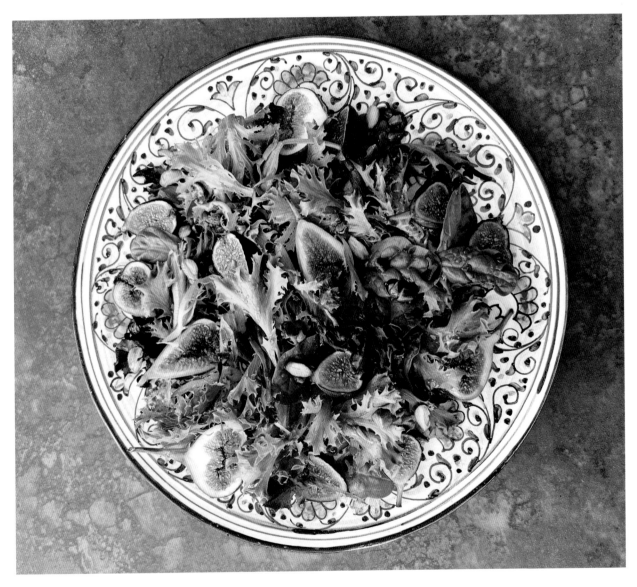

LENTIL SOUP WITH FRESH HERBS AND OLIVE OIL

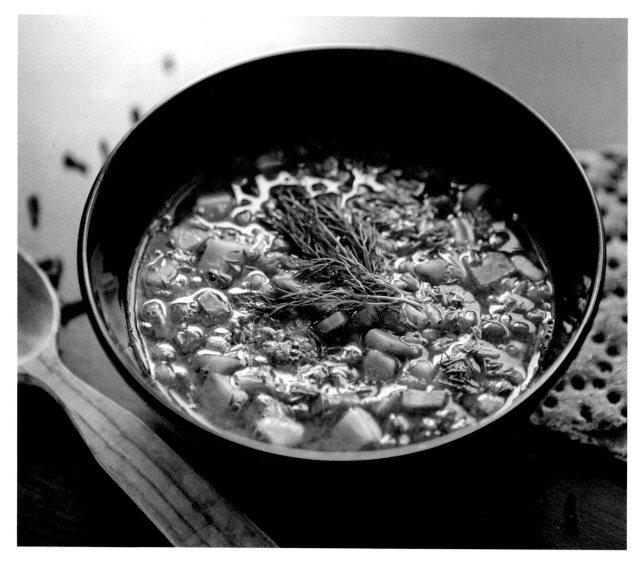

Lentil soup is a staple on Ikaria; it's full of protein, good fats, and tons of flavor. This one relies on the best quality olive oil to finish. Feel free to use whatever herbs you have on hand.

Serves 8

¼ cup (60 ml) Greek olive oil

1 cup (142 g) chopped yellow onion

1 cup (142 g) peeled and chopped carrots

1 cup (142 g) chopped celery

2 cups (384 g) brown or green lentils

4 cloves garlic, minced

5 cups (1.2 L) water

2 cups (500 g) tomato sauce

1 bay leaf

¾ teaspoon sea salt

½ teaspoon freshly ground black pepper

1 cup (12 g) mixed fresh herbs (dill, mint, parsley, thyme, basil), coarsely chopped

Extra-virgin olive oil for drizzling

1. Add the olive oil to a large Dutch oven over medium heat.

2. Once hot, add the onion, carrots, and celery, and sauté, stirring occasionally, for 5 to 7 minutes, or until tender and lightly browned.

3. Stir in the lentils and garlic, coating in the olive oil.

4. Add the water, tomato sauce, and bay leaf. Stir and turn the heat up to medium-high. Bring to a boil.

5. Reduce the heat to medium-low and simmer, stirring occasionally, for 25 to 30 minutes, or until the lentils are tender and thickened.

6. Remove from heat, remove bay leaf, and season with salt and pepper.

7. To serve, ladle into bowls, sprinkle with fresh herbs, and drizzle with extra-virgin olive oil.

This dish is the perfect use of fresh, just–picked vegetables, right out of the garden. On Ikaria, the stars of this dish are the olive oil and the summer vegetables, but you may substitute whatever vegetables are in season for you. Soufiko is similar to French ratatouille but includes potatoes. The beauty of this dish is in the layering; take a little extra time to layer the veggies, and the presentation will be well worth it!

Serves 8

½ cup (120 ml) Greek extra–virgin olive oil, divided

2 medium eggplants, sliced in rounds ¼ inch thick

2 sweet onions, sliced in rounds ¼ inch thick

2 medium zucchini, sliced in rounds ¼ inch thick

2 russet potatoes, peeled and sliced in rounds ¼ inch thick

2 red or yellow bell peppers, sliced into thin strips

4 cloves garlic, minced

2 teaspoons (5 g) sea salt

4 Roma tomatoes, coarsely chopped

2 tablespoons (2 g) fresh Greek marjoram or oregano, chopped

1. Preheat the oven 375˚F (190˚C, or gas mark 5).

2. In a large heavy-bottomed sauté pan, heat 2 tablespoons (30 ml) of the olive oil over medium heat.

3. Once hot, add the sliced eggplant and cook 3 minutes per side, or until browned and tender. Transfer to a plate (do not drain).

4. Add another 1 tablespoon (15 ml) olive oil to the pan. When hot, add the onions and sauté for 5 minutes total, or until lightly browned and tender. Transfer to the plate with the eggplant.

5. Add 1 more tablespoon (15 ml) of olive oil. Once hot, add the zucchini and sauté on each side for 3 minutes, or until lightly browned and tender. Transfer to the plate with the eggplant and onions. Remove the pan from the heat.

6. In the same sauté pan, arrange the eggplant, onions, zucchini, potatoes, and bell peppers in layers. (Or, for an incredible presentation, alternate vegetables in a concentric circle starting in the middle and working your way out to the edges of a gratin dish.)

7. Sprinkle with the minced garlic and sea salt. Top with the chopped tomatoes, drizzle with the remaining olive oil and sprinkle with fresh oregano.

8. Cover with a tight-fitting lid or foil and transfer to the oven.

9. Bake for 20 to 30 minutes, or until the potatoes are tender and the tomatoes have made a sauce.

10. Serve hot or at room temperature.

SOUFIKO (IKARIAN RATATOUILLE)

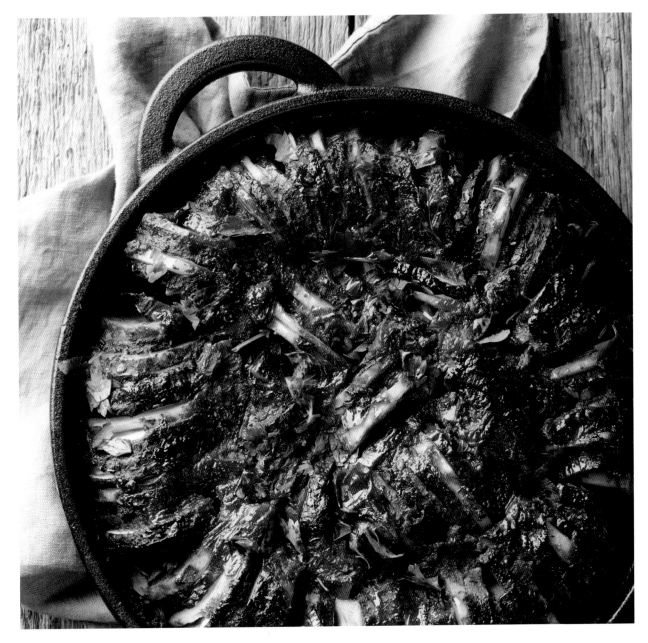

WILTED GREENS WITH GRILLED FENNEL, SLOW-ROASTED TOMATOES, AND LENTILS

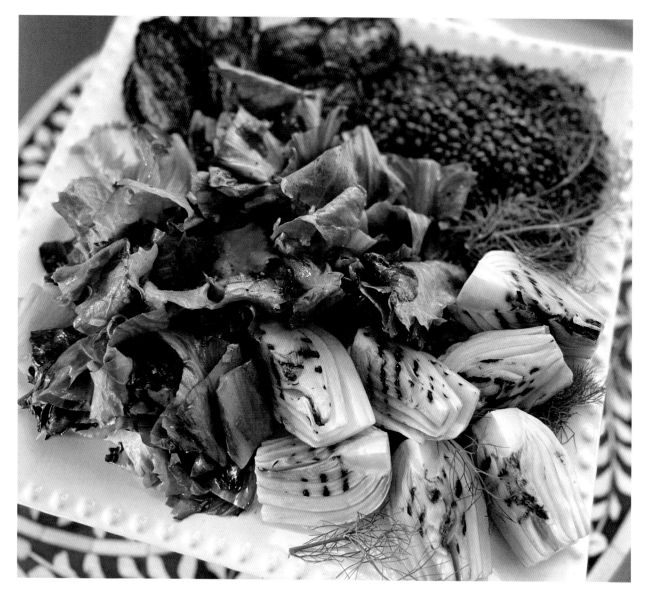

The flavors of this salad are exquisite. It does take a little bit of time to get all the ingredients prepared, but they can each be made 3 to 4 days in advance and put together right before serving. I love this dish made with escarole, but any bitter green would work well, so switch it up with radicchio or arugula.

Serves 4

4 Roma tomatoes, cut lengthwise

1 tablespoon (15 ml) olive oil

1 teaspoon sugar

½ teaspoon sea salt

2 cups (470 ml) water

½ cup (96 g) green lentils

2 bulbs fennel

½ cup (120 ml) Greek extra-virgin olive oil

¼ cup (30 g) minced shallot

2 cloves garlic, minced

¼ cup (60 ml) fresh orange juice

2 tablespoons (43 g) raw honey

2 tablespoons (30 g) Dijon mustard

6 cups (6 oz [170 g]) coarsely chopped escarole or other bitter greens

½ teaspoon sea salt

¼ teaspoon freshly ground black pepper

1. Preheat the oven to 300°F (150°C, or gas mark 2). Line a baking sheet with parchment paper and set a rack on top.

2. Add the tomatoes to a large bowl, drizzle with the olive oil, sugar, and sea salt. Toss to coat.

3. Arrange the tomatoes cut side up on the prepared baking sheet. Transfer to the oven and roast for 2 hours. Remove from heat and allow to cool.

4. In a small saucepan over medium-high heat, add the water and lentils. Bring to a boil, reduce the heat to low, and simmer for 17 to 20 minutes, or until tender but not mushy. Remove from heat, drain any remaining water, and allow to cool.

5. While the lentils cook, prepare the fennel by cutting the tops off the bulbs (reserve the fennel fronds). Remove any outside tough parts and cut into quarters through the stem.

6. Preheat a grill pan over medium-high heat. Add the fennel and grill for 2 to 3 minutes on each side, or until lightly charred and tender. Remove from heat. Once cool, slice into ½-inch slices.

7. In a large heavy-bottomed pan, heat the extra-virgin olive oil over medium heat. Add the shallot and garlic and sauté for 1 minute. Whisk in the orange juice, honey, and mustard.

8. Add the escarole to the dressing and using a whisk, toss to coat.

9. To serve, arrange the room-temperature tomatoes, fennel, and lentils on a large platter. Top with the slightly wilted greens and any remaining dressing. Season with salt and pepper, and garnish with reserved fennel fronds, if desired. Serve immediately.

This soup is a winter favorite on Ikaria: nourishing, flavorful, fiber rich, and filling on a cold day. I prefer to puree a little of the soup and add it back in for a silkier texture, but if you like a chunkier soup, you can skip that step.

Serves 8

1 pound (454 g) dried chickpeas, soaked overnight in cool water (8 to 12 hours)

6 cups (1.4 L) water

½ cup (120 ml) Greek extra-virgin olive oil

1½ cups (213 g) chopped red onion

8 cloves garlic, minced

2 teaspoons (3 g) dried oregano

1 bay leaf

½ cup (120 ml) fresh lemon juice

2 tablespoons (4 g) lemon zest

1 teaspoon sea salt

½ teaspoon freshly ground black pepper

1 cup (12 g) mixed fresh herbs (oregano, dill, parsley, and mint), coarsely chopped

Crushed red pepper flakes (optional)

1. Drain and rinse the soaked chickpeas with cold water. Transfer to a large pot, cover with cold water, and bring to a boil over high heat. Boil for 15 minutes.

2. Drain the chickpeas one more time, rinse, and then return them to the large pot and cover with 6 cups (1.4 L) cold water. Add the olive oil, red onion, garlic, oregano, and bay leaf. Bring to a boil, reduce heat to medium-low, and simmer for 1½ to 2 hours, or until tender. Remove from heat and remove the bay leaf.

3. If you wish to have a creamier soup, transfer 1 cup (196 g) of the chickpeas to a high-powered blender and blend on high until smooth and creamy. Add back to the soup pot and stir to incorporate.

4. Add the lemon juice and zest, and season with salt and pepper.

5. To serve, ladle into bowls and top with the mixed herbs and red pepper flakes, if desired.

CHICKPEA SOUP WITH GARLIC, LEMON, AND HERBS

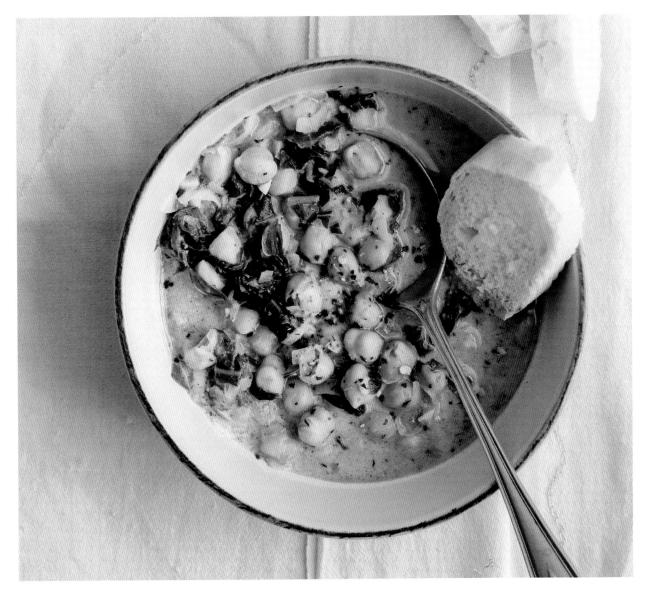

WILD GREENS POT PIE

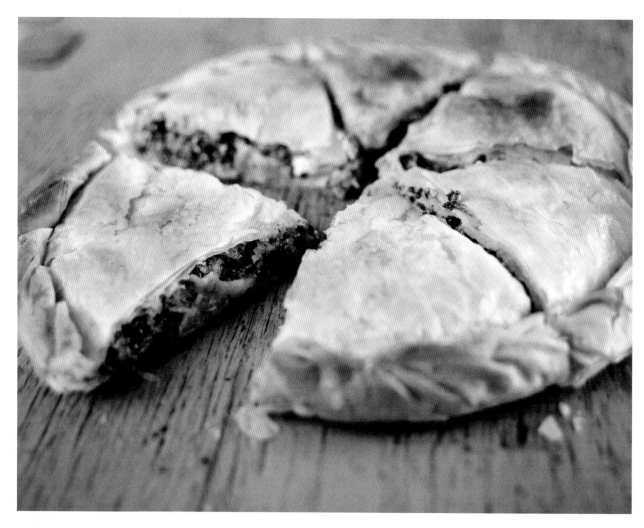

This spectacular dish is light, crispy, and full of wild greens. If you can't find dandelion greens (often available at farmers' markets), swap them out for other greens, or use all spinach.

Serves 8

8 cups (4 oz [114 g]) mixed wild greens (dandelion, arugula, spinach, Swiss chard), finely chopped

1 cup (12 g) mixed tender herbs (dill, parsley, chervil, chives), finely chopped

½ cup (120 ml) Greek olive oil, divided

1½ teaspoons (4 g) sea salt

½ teaspoon freshly ground black pepper

½ cup (32 g) chopped scallions

2 cloves garlic, minced

1 tablespoon (2 g) lemon zest

1 tablespoon (15 ml) fresh lemon juice

8 sheets phyllo dough, thawed

1. Preheat the oven to 400°F (200°C, or gas mark 6). Brush a 9-inch (23-cm) glass pie plate with olive oil. Set aside.

2. In a large bowl, combine the chopped greens, chopped herbs, and ¼ cup (60 ml) of the olive oil, salt, and pepper. Massage together to gently wilt the greens, then set aside.

3. In a small sauté pan over medium heat, add 1 tablespoon (15 ml) of the olive oil. Once warm, add the scallions and garlic and sauté for 1 minute. Add to the wilted greens and stir to wilt the greens even further.

4. Add in the lemon zest and juice and stir to combine.

5. To assemble the pie, unroll the thawed phyllo dough and, while you are working, keep it covered with a moist and clean kitchen towel. Working with 1 sheet at a time, lay the phyllo dough so that it is centered in the prepared pie plate, draping excess dough over the rim of the plate. Brush thoroughly with about 1 teaspoon olive oil. Repeat with 3 more phyllo sheets, for 4 total, brushing with oil in between each layer.

6. Add the greens mixture to the phyllo-lined pie.

7. Top the pie with 4 more layers of phyllo, brushing with oil in between each layer and tucking the dough around the greens mixture. Fold the overlapping phyllo and roll around the edges to make a nice edge.

8. Score the phyllo dough into 8 even sections, like you'd cut a pie. This will make it easier to cut once it is baked.

9. Transfer to the oven and bake for 35 to 45 minutes, or until golden brown and puffed. Allow to sit for 10 minutes before sliding out from the pie plate and slicing.

This light soup is a perfect combination of wilted greens, orzo, and Greek olive oil. It is light and refreshing and perfect in both the summer and winter months.

Serves 8

2 tablespoons (30 ml) Greek olive oil

1 cup (142 g) chopped onion

4 cloves garlic, minced

2 quarts (1.9 L) vegetable broth

1½ cups (270 g) orzo

½ cup (120 ml) fresh lemon juice

⅓ cup (74 g) tahini

4 cups (2 oz [57 g]) mixed greens (spinach, chard, and kale), coarsely chopped

½ cup (8 g) dill, chopped

¾ teaspoon sea salt

½ teaspoon freshly ground black pepper

1. Heat the oil in a large Dutch oven over medium heat. Add the onion and sauté for 5 minutes, or until wilted and translucent.

2. Stir in the garlic and cook for 30 seconds, or until fragrant.

3. Add the broth and bring to a boil over medium-high heat. Add the orzo, reduce the heat to medium-low, and simmer for 8 minutes, or until the orzo is tender.

4. Remove from heat, whisk in the lemon juice and tahini until combined.

5. Add in the chopped greens and stir until wilted.

6. Stir in the dill, and season with salt and pepper.

OLIVE OIL, ORZO, AND WILD GREENS SOUP

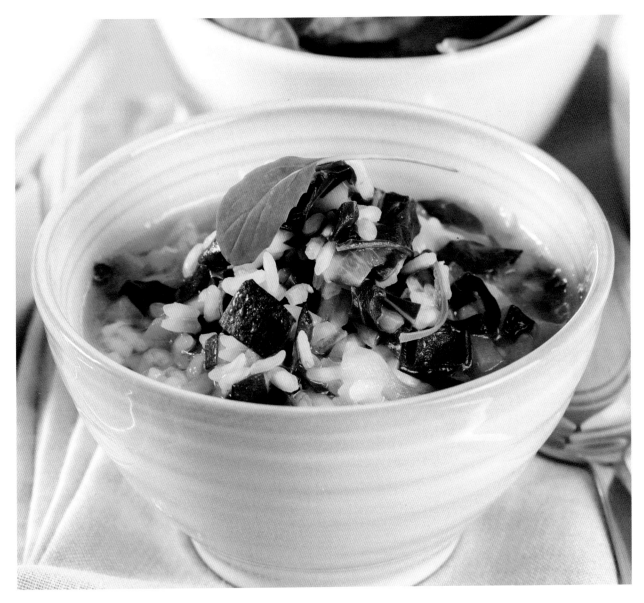

POTATO-HERB SALAD WITH LEMON VINAIGRETTE

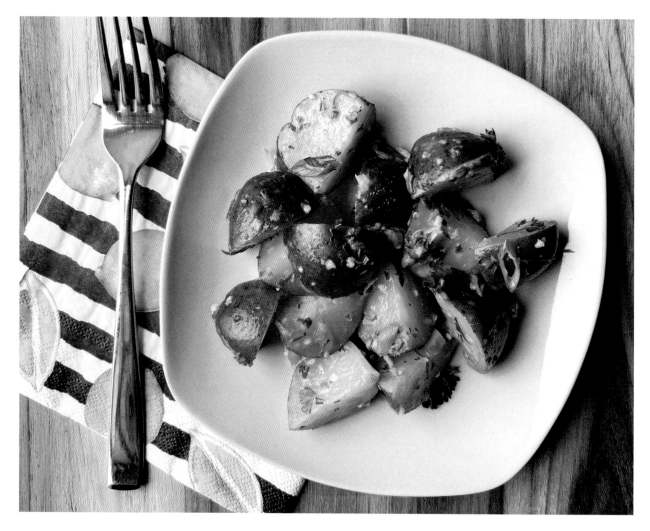

This is a light and fresh potato salad made with olive oil and herbs. Feel free to change the herbs to your liking and depending on what you're serving this dish alongside.

Serves 4 to 6

2 pounds (907 g) small red potatoes, scrubbed and quartered

1 tablespoon (8 g) sea salt

¼ cup (60 ml) Greek extra-virgin olive oil

½ cup (6 g) lightly packed fresh flat-leaf parsley, coarsely chopped, divided

½ cup (32 g) coarsely chopped scallions, divided

2 tablespoons (30 ml) fresh lemon juice

2 teaspoons (10 g) Dijon mustard

2 cloves garlic, minced

½ teaspoon freshly ground black pepper

½ cup (71 g) finely chopped celery

1. In a large pot or Dutch oven, add the potatoes and salt and cover with cold water. Bring to a boil over medium-high heat, then reduce heat to medium and cook until the potatoes can be pierced with a paring knife that pulls out easily, 8 to 10 minutes.

2. Reserve ½ cup (120 ml) of the cooking liquid, then drain the remaining liquid from the potatoes.

3. Transfer the potatoes to a large bowl.

4. In the bowl of a food processor or blender, add the olive oil, ⅓ cup (5 g) of the parsley, ⅓ cup (21 g) of the scallions, lemon juice, mustard, garlic, and pepper. Blend or puree on high until the herbs are finely chopped. With the motor running, add in ¼ cup (60 ml) of the reserved liquid. If still too thick, add a little bit more.

5. Pour the dressing over the cooked potatoes and toss to coat. Stir in the remaining parsley and scallions and the celery to incorporate.

6. Serve cold or at room temperature.

Olive oil–cornmeal cakes are truly divine, and this one—pared with dried fruit—is rustic and delicious. The dense texture is made a little lighter with the addition of Greek yogurt, but it is otherwise plant-based. This cake is enjoyed on Ikaria as a breakfast or dessert.

Serves 8

2 cups (304 g) coarse cornmeal

¼ cup (53 g) sugar

1 tablespoon (14 g) baking powder

½ teaspoon baking soda

½ teaspoon kosher salt

¾ cup (180 ml) fresh orange juice

½ cup (120 ml) Greek extra-virgin olive oil

½ cup (128 g) plain Greek yogurt

½ cup (75 g) golden raisins

½ cup (75 g) dried figs, chopped

¼ cup (32 g) dried apricots, chopped

¼ cup (43 g) candied orange peel, chopped

2 tablespoons (4 g) orange zest

1 cup (235 ml) hot water

½ cup (170 g) Greek honey

1. Preheat the oven to 375°F (190°C, or gas mark 5). Brush a deep-dish pie plate with olive oil. Set aside.

2. In a medium bowl, whisk together the cornmeal, sugar, baking powder, baking soda, and salt.

3. In another bowl, whisk together the orange juice, olive oil, and yogurt.

4. Add the cornmeal mixture to the wet mixture and whisk until combined.

5. Gently fold in the raisins, figs, apricots, candied orange peel, and orange zest. Fold until just combined.

6. Spoon the batter into the prepared pie plate and transfer to the oven. Bake for 40 minutes, or until a toothpick inserted in the center comes out clean.

7. While the cake is baking, make the syrup. In a medium saucepan over low heat, add the water and honey. Bring to a simmer and cook for 8 minutes. Remove from heat.

8. When the cake is done baking, prick it all over with a fork. Pour the syrup over the top and allow to cool and absorb the syrup. Cool completely before slicing.

CORNMEAL CAKE WITH DRIED FRUIT AND OLIVE OIL

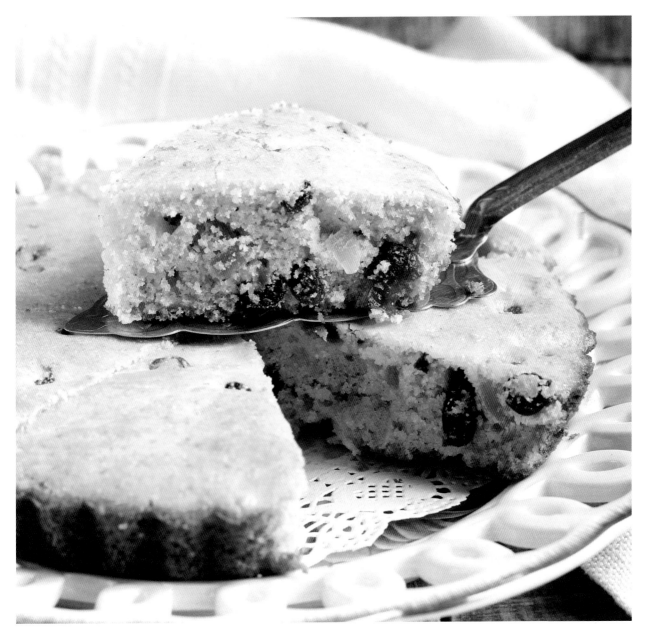

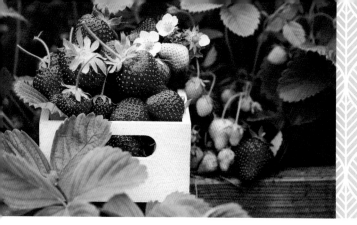

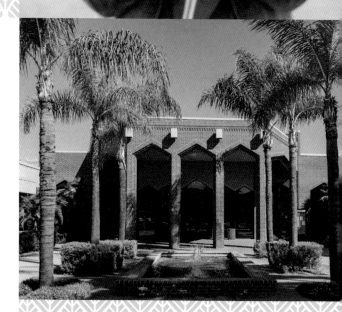

CHAPTER 3

LOMA LINDA, CALIFORNIA

Loma Linda, California, translates to "Beautiful Hill," and is home to 9,000 Seventh-day Adventists who, on average, live about a decade longer than people in any other area of the United States. This group leads a vegetarian, alcohol-free, and smoke-free life and maintains an active lifestyle. The reason attributed to their longevity is that they treat their bodies as a temple, and they believe that we are meant to eat vegetables, not kill animals for food. This vegetarian and health-minded community has a wealth of research knowledge, and their studies from the Loma Linda University Medical University aid in breakthroughs about preventative medicine, healthy eating, and longevity.

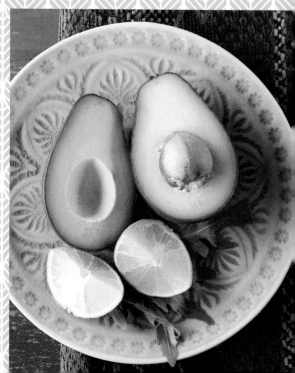

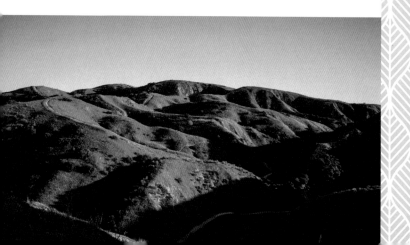

A Day in the Life

Like most of Southern California, Loma Linda boasts year-round sunshine with near perfect temperatures. This climate makes it ideal for a healthy lifestyle of outdoor living. Most people tend to slow down when retired, but the older residents of Loma Linda do anything but that. This group of religious and health-minded people tend to start the day at dawn with a nutritious breakfast of whole grains. A favorite such as overnight chia pudding or oatmeal with nuts, hemp seeds, and fruit is a perfect start to the day. Homemade bread, homemade jams, and fresh fruit are also regular breakfast offerings. Following breakfast, a hike through the breathtaking hills around Loma Linda is the perfect way to watch the sunrise and get up to 12 miles of exercise before a lot of us have even begun the day.

Now that the sun has risen and morning exercise done, a morning worship and a crossword puzzle keep the spirits high and the mind sharp. Daily devotion is a part of this community's life and is what gives the older residents purpose. This faith-based group devotes most of their lives to living spiritually and with meaning, to reducing stress in their daily lives, and to creating a sustainable existence.

Loma Linda residents make sure that every moment of their lives is spent sharing with the community, being a light for those around them, and offering prayers and words of encouragement to all. Volunteering is a huge part of daily life and can look like food or clothing drives, working in public offices, or aiding in the retirement communities.

Loma Lindans believe that their rich diversity, with people and cultures coming from everywhere in the world to be a part of their Seventh-day Adventist community, is what makes this particular place such a strong and faith-filled one. The community center is a place where everyone comes together, and lunch is one of those bustling times. Lunch is simple with fresh salads, soups or stews, and sandwiches. The food is unadorned yet flavorful, and the company is strong and filled with laughter, faith, and so much love. A trip to the grocery store shows that even though the Seventh-day Adventists comprise only about one-third of the population of Loma Linda, their ideals have spread further: bin after bin of dried nuts, seeds, beans, and legumes.... and no meat section! There are honor systems in place to purchase the fresh fruit and vegetables from the local stands.

Sabbath every Saturday is a time where everyone in the community comes together to worship and, of course, eat. It's like one huge potluck, everyone contributing a dish that is locally grown, seasonal, and delicious. A potluck item might be the famous layered taco salad or a bean and vegetable stew. After outdoor and indoor exercising, eating local and seasonal vegetarian food, and participating in family, faith, and devotion, the day ends in Loma Linda with a family dinner, studies, worship, and the knowledge that their purpose in life is being fulfilled and that a full night's rest is what is needed to start the journey all over again tomorrow.

The Food of Loma Linda

Loma Linda, California, is perhaps the healthiest community in the United States. It all boils down to its population of Seventh-day Adventists. This tight-knit community is one based on faith, trust, purpose, unity, and a clean, plant-rich diet. Here are some of the staples that make up the Loma Lindan cuisine and their health benefits.

AVOCADOS The mighty avocado! This fruit, found in abundance in California, is a nutritional dynamite, chock full of vitamins C, E, K, and B_6, as well as niacin, folate, riboflavin, pantothenic acid, magnesium, and potassium. They are also a good source of omega-3 fatty acids, beta carotene, and lutein. This healthy fat keeps us feeling satiated, as well as being super beneficial for eye health. The fatty acids in avocados help maintain a healthy blood pressure and help to keep our heart healthy.

NUTS Nuts are an integral part of the Loma Linda cuisine. Containing fiber, vitamin E, magnesium, phosphorus, copper, manganese, and selenium, nuts are an excellent source of protein and a perfect addition to a well-balanced diet. They are loaded with antioxidants, which help to fight and neutralize free radicals that may increase the risk of disease. Nuts have also been shown to help lower "bad" LDL cholesterol and help increase "good" HDL cholesterol. Research has further shown that nuts have a positive effect on reducing inflammation, are a great prebiotic for gut health, and help to reduce the risk of heart disease and stroke.

BEANS Another great source of plant-based protein and fiber, beans are wonderful at helping to control your appetite and promoting gut health. These high-antioxidant pulses are a great source of folate, zinc, and magnesium. They have been shown to aid in heart health, help control diabetes, and help maintain a healthy weight.

OATS Oats are a naturally gluten free whole grain and a good source of manganese, phosphorus, magnesium, copper, iron, zinc, folate, vitamin B_1, and vitamin B_6. Oatmeal has been shown to aid in weight loss by keeping us feeling satisfied, lowering fat and carbohydrate absorption, and stabilizing blood glucose levels; it can also help lower the risk of heart disease. One of the most powerful compounds found in oatmeal is an antioxidant called avenanthramides. This newly researched compound has been shown to help dilate blood vessels, which increases blood flow and helps lower blood pressure. Promoting gut health, heart health, blood sugar control, weight loss, skin health, and asthma control are just a few of the amazing qualities of this simple grain.

CAULIFLOWER Cauliflower is part of the cruciferous family and can be found in white, orange, purple, and green. This high-fiber vegetable also contains a lot of water, meaning it can keep you hydrated. One of the main substances found in cauliflower is called glucosinolates. These cancer fighting compounds are created when you chew and digest cauliflower, and they help to protect cells from damage and have anti-inflammatory, antiviral, and antibacterial properties. Cauliflower is also a great source of vitamin C and a good source of vitamin K, calcium, iron, potassium, and magnesium.

SPROUTED GRAINS These whole grains have more readily available vitamins and minerals than their unsprouted counterparts. They must be eaten in controlled ways because of the potential for

bacterial growth, but when eaten in baked goods, the benefits are incredible. When grains are sprouted or germinated, some of the starch is broken down, which makes their nutrient content higher. This process also breaks down a phytic acid found in grains called phytate. Phytate normally decreases absorption of vitamins and minerals in the body, but with sprouted grains the opposite (a higher absorption rate) is true. Folate, iron, vitamin C, zinc, magnesium, and protein are some of the more easily digestible nutrients found in sprouted grains. Look for sprouted-grain products in the natural foods sections of grocery stores.

SEEDS These mighty little superfoods at the outset of life contain all the nutrients essential for growing a mature healthy adult plant. They offer the same benefits to our bodies as well. Some of the most common seeds are flax, chia, pumpkin, sunflower, poppy, sesame, and psyllium, all of which contain omega-3 fatty acids, vitamin E, and B vitamins. These pack high-quality protein, heart-healthy fats, and essential vitamins and minerals useful for boosting immune, hormonal, and cardiovascular health.

KALE This leafy green cruciferous veggie in the cabbage family is well known for its health benefits. This nutrient-dense vegetable is high in vitamins A, K, C, and B_6, manganese, calcium, copper, potassium, and magnesium, and it's a good source of vitamins B_1, B_2, B_3, iron, and phosphorus. Kale also contains the omega-3 fatty acid called alpha-linolenic acid and the amazing compound quercetin. This compound has been shown to have powerful heart protection and has blood pressure–lowering, anti-inflammatory,

antiviral, antidepressant, and anticancer effects! Among kale's other impressive claims, collagen production, cholesterol lowering, heart protecting, osteoporosis preventing, cancer fighting, and eye protection are some of the more impressive ones.

TOMATOES Tomatoes, like avocados, are a staple of Californian cuisine. When used raw, the vitamin C content of a tomato is more present; when cooked, the lycopene content increases. When eaten in season, this beautiful, flavorful fruit has been shown to protect eyes; lower LDL ("bad") cholesterol and blood pressure; protect against lung, stomach, and prostate cancers; and fight inflammation.

ONIONS, GARLIC, PEPPERS Often used together as a flavorful base for Loma Lindan cuisine, onions, garlic, and peppers are a perfect foundation of health and nutrition. Quercetin, a powerful antioxidant and cancer-attacking agent, is known as an antiviral, anti-inflammatory, and anticancer aid. Together, these three also have incredible respiratory healing properties. The sulfuric compounds in onions and garlic, especially, help prevent inflammation, fight mucus, and act as a natural expectorant.

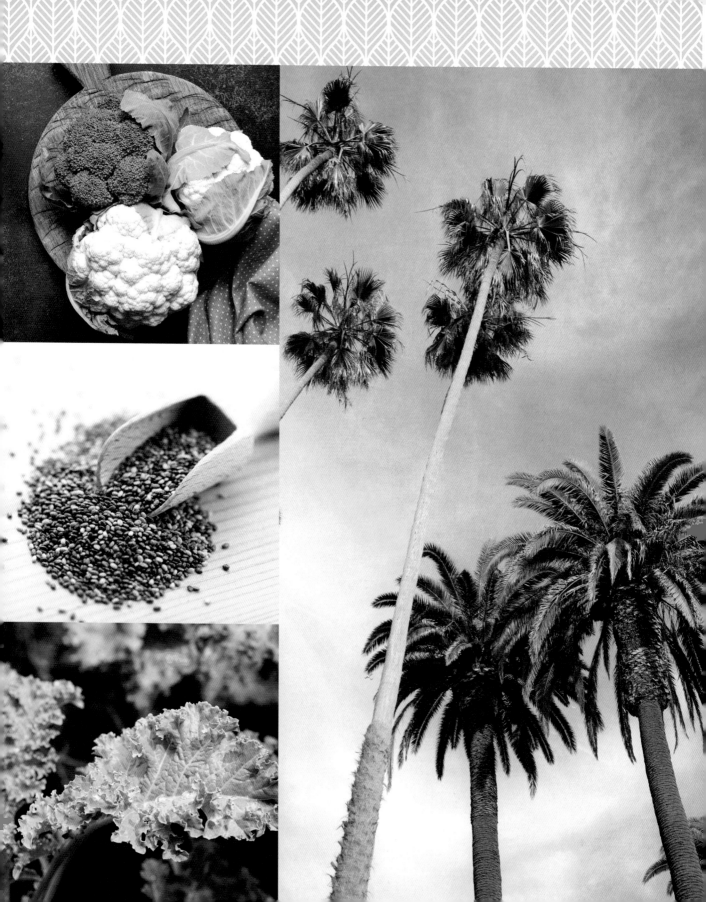

The Recipes of Loma Linda

THE BEST OVERNIGHT CHIA PUDDING

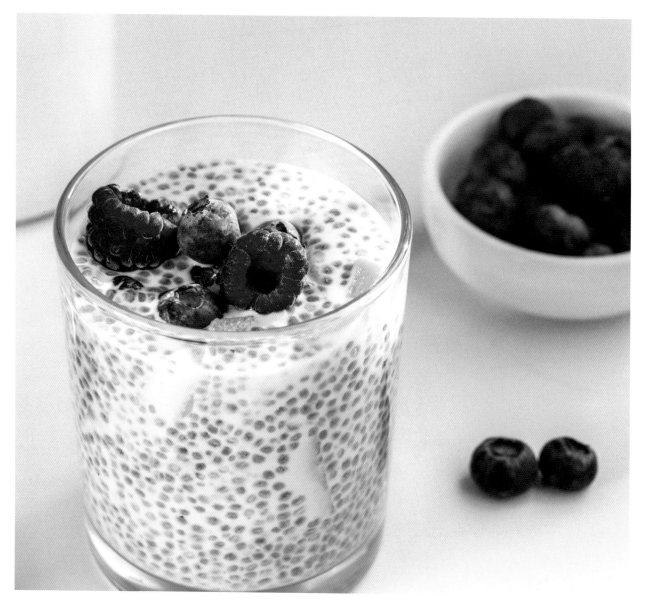

Chia pudding is such an easy and nutritious breakfast, snack, or dessert. Containing healthy fats, protein, and fiber, seeds are such an important part of the Loma Linda lifestyle. This pudding takes about 5 minutes to make and is ready for when you wake up; all you have to do is give it a good shake. The flavor possibilities are endless, so make this to your liking.

Serves 2

PUDDING:

1 cup (235 ml) almond or oat milk

4 tablespoons (40 g) sprouted chia seeds

2 teaspoons (10 ml) maple syrup

1 teaspoon vanilla extract

TOPPINGS:

¼ cup (20 g) shredded toasted coconut

¼ cup (29 g) slivered almonds, toasted (see page 31)

¼ cup (38 g) quartered fresh strawberries

¼ cup (38 g) fresh blueberries and/or raspberries

1. To make the puddings, start with two clean, 12-ounce (355-ml) glass jars with tight-fitting lids.

2. Divide the milk, chia seeds, maple syrup, and vanilla between the jars. Cover with the lid, and shake the container until all the chia seeds are dispersed and stay that way when you stop shaking.

3. Transfer to the refrigerator and allow to sit overnight.

4. When ready to eat, add toppings, as desired, and enjoy immediately or take it to go.

A smoothie is an incredible way to pack vitamins, minerals, antioxidants, good fats, and protein into one simple drink. This smoothie is one that utilizes nut butter, flax, fresh greens and avocado, and fresh and frozen fruit. Feel free to make combinations that you love!

Serves 2

2 cups (1 oz [29 g]) fresh baby spinach or chopped kale

2 peeled and sliced frozen bananas

1 ripe avocado, peeled and pitted

4 cups (592 g) frozen or fresh blueberries

2 tablespoons (13 g) ground flaxseed

2 tablespoons (32 g) almond or peanut butter

½ teaspoon ground cinnamon

1 cup (235 ml) unsweetened vanilla nut or oat milk

1. Place all ingredients in the blender in the order they are listed.

2. Blend on high until smooth and creamy. Divide between glasses and enjoy.

A SMOOTHIE A DAY

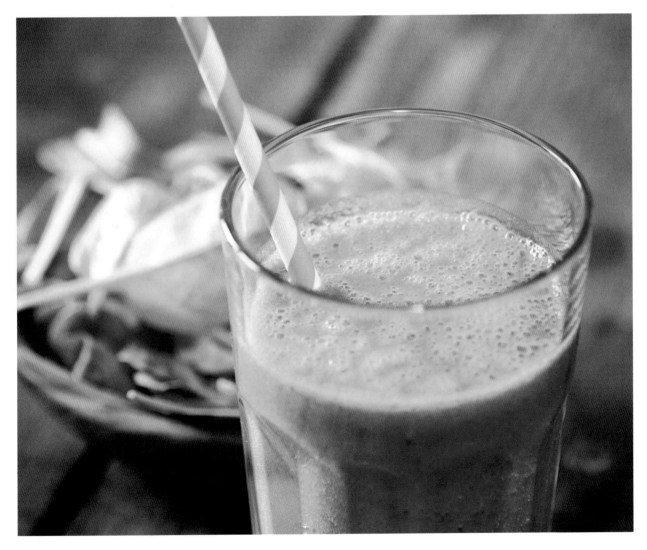

HOMEMADE GRANOLA AND FRUIT PARFAITS

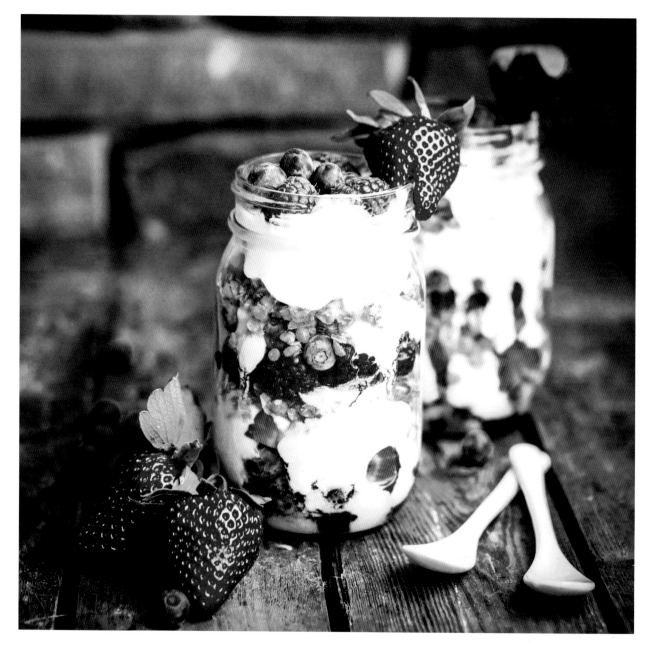

This fruit parfait is an incredible and easy-to-pull-together breakfast. You can make the granola ahead of time and once cool, store it in an airtight container in the fridge for up to 3 weeks. Choose fruit that is in season and switch it up during the seasons. Make these the night before for a very quick and healthy breakfast.

Serves 2

GRANOLA:

2 cups (284 g) almonds, chopped

1 cup (128 g) pecans, chopped

1 cup (128 g) walnuts, chopped

1 cup (120 g) pepitas

1 cup (140 g) sunflower seeds

¾ cup (60 g) unsweetened shredded coconut

¾ cup (86 g) dried cranberries

¼ cup (36 g) sesame seeds

¼ cup (26 g) ground flaxseeds

½ teaspoon ground cloves

½ teaspoon ground cinnamon

½ teaspoon kosher salt

½ cup (120 ml) maple syrup or (170 g) honey

6 tablespoons (90 ml) coconut oil, melted

1 teaspoon vanilla extract

PARFAIT:

1 cup (140 g) granola

1 cup (256 g) plain Greek yogurt, plant-based or regular

1 cup (150 g) mixed berries (strawberries, blackberries, blueberries, raspberries)

1. To make the granola: Preheat the oven to 275°F (135°C, or gas mark 1). Line 2 baking sheets with parchment paper and set aside.

2. In a large bowl, add the nuts, seeds, dried fruit, and spices, and stir to combine.

3. In a medium bowl, add the maple syrup, coconut oil, and vanilla, whisking to combine.

4. Pour the wet ingredients over the dry and toss to coat.

5. Arrange on the 2 prepared baking sheets and transfer to the oven.

6. Bake for 45 to 60 minutes, stirring every 15 minutes to avoid burning.

7. Once the granola is golden brown, remove from the oven and allow to cool completely. This recipe makes about 8 cups (1.1 kg).

8. To make the parfaits: Spoon ¼ cup (35 g) granola into a parfait glass or other glass. Top with ¼ cup (35 g) yogurt, ¼ cup (38 g) fruit, and repeat the process again ending with fruit. Repeat for a second parfait.

Serves 4

TAHINI DRESSING:

¼ cup (56 g) tahini

¼ cup (60 ml) water

1 tablespoon (15 ml) sherry vinegar

1 tablespoon (14 ml) maple syrup

2 teaspoons (10 ml) chili sauce

½ teaspoon kosher salt

¼ teaspoon ground turmeric

BOWLS:

¼ cup (60 ml) olive oil

2 teaspoons (5 g) smoked paprika

2 teaspoons (5 g) garlic powder

1 teaspoon ground cumin

1 teaspoon kosher salt

6 cups (600 g) cauliflower florets

3 medium or 2 large carrots, peeled and cut into
   1-inch pieces (about 1½ cups)

1 large white yam, peeled and cut into 1-inch pieces
   (about 1½ cups)

½ pound (227 g) Brussels sprouts, trimmed and cut
   in half (about 1 cup)

2 cups (470 ml) vegetable broth

1 cup (180 g) sprouted dry quinoa

1 tablespoon (15 ml) avocado oil

4 cups (80 g) chopped kale

2 tablespoons (30 ml) tamari

2 avocados, sliced

1. To make the tahini dressing: Combine the tahini,
    water, vinegar, maple syrup, chili sauce, salt, and
    turmeric in a small bowl. Whisk until smooth and
    creamy. Set aside.

2. To make the bowls: Preheat the oven to 425°F
    (220°C, or gas mark 7). Line 2 baking sheets with
    parchment paper and set aside.

3. In a small bowl, whisk together the olive oil,
    smoked paprika, garlic powder, cumin, and salt.

4. In a large bowl, add the cauliflower and one-
    third of the olive oil mixture. Toss to coat.
    Arrange on one of the prepared baking sheets.
    In the same bowl, add the carrots and yams and
    another one-third of the olive oil mixture. Toss
    to coat and arrange on one-half of the second
    baking sheet. Lastly, add the Brussels sprouts
    and the rest of the oil mixture. Toss to coat and
    arrange on the other half of the baking sheet.

5. Transfer both baking sheets to the oven and
    roast for 25 to 30 minutes, tossing halfway
    through roasting, or until the vegetables are
    tender, crisp, and caramelized.

6. While the vegetables roast, make the quinoa.
    Add the vegetable broth and quinoa to a
    medium saucepan over medium-high heat.
    Bring to a boil, reduce heat, cover, and gently
    simmer for 10 to 12 minutes, until the quinoa is
    light and fluffy, all the broth is absorbed, and the
    kernels pop open. Turn off the heat and allow
    to sit for 5 minutes. Remove lid and fluff quinoa
    with a fork. Set aside.

7. In a large sauté pan with a tight-fitting lid, heat
    the avocado oil over medium heat. Add the kale
    and cover to steam for 3 to 5 minutes. Remove
    the lid, turn off the heat, stir, and season with
    the tamari.

8. To assemble a bowl, put one-quarter of the
    quinoa on the bottom. Top with one-quarter of
    the kale and one-quarter of the roasted veggies.
    Add half of a sliced avocado and drizzle with the
    tahini dressing.

CALIFORNIA VEGGIE BOWL WITH TAHINI DRESSING

The veggie bowl is a quintessential California staple. It's best when seasonal vegetables are utilized for a simple yet delicious meal. This bowl showcases fall vegetables, but switch it up and enjoy it year round. You can also play with the grain you use; brown rice, quinoa, farro, or even barley would make an excellent base.

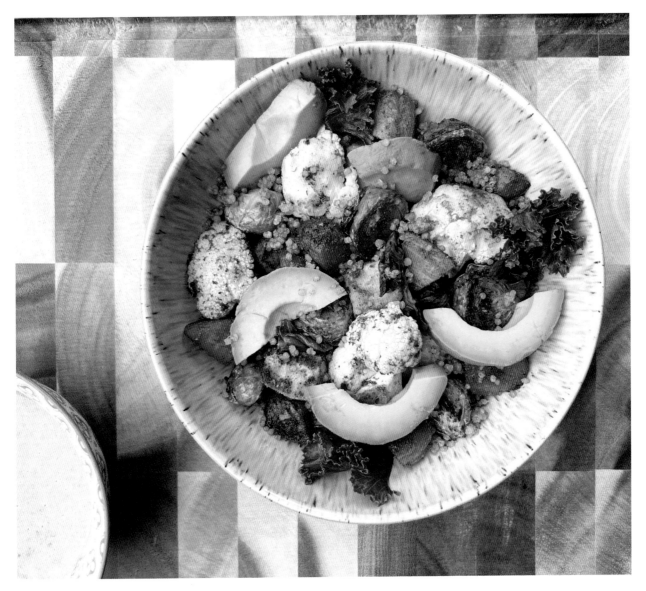

SLOW COOKER BEAN AND VEGETABLE SOUP

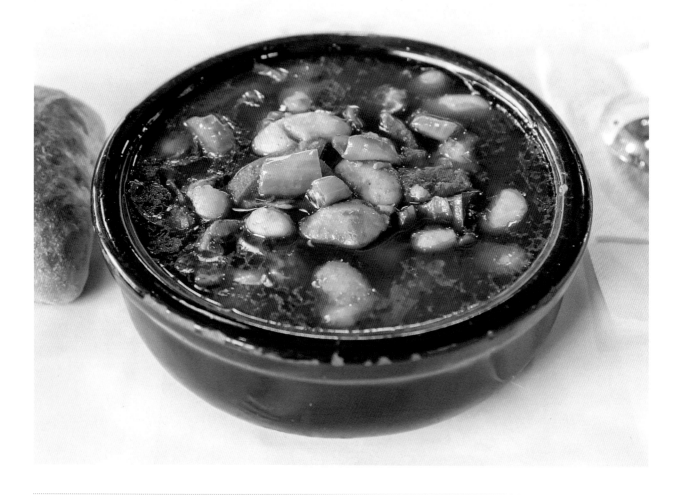

The slow cooker is often used to create healthy and nutritious kitchen creations. This soup has an extra step of soaking the beans the night before, but that's the hardest part! The rest of this soup comes together quickly and without much effort. If you don't have a slow cooker, you may cook this soup on low heat on the stove until the beans are tender.

Serves 8 to 12

1 pound (454 g) great northern beans, soaked overnight in cool water (8 to 12 hours)

2 cups (284 g) peeled and chopped carrots

2 cups (284 g) chopped celery

2 cups (284 g) chopped sweet onion

6 ounces (170 g) cremini mushrooms, sliced (about 1½ cups)

1 cup (242 g) canned diced tomatoes, with their juice

2 tablespoons (28 g) minced garlic

2 tablespoons (33 g) tomato paste

1 tablespoon (4 g) Italian seasoning

1 quart (946 ml) vegetable broth

2 cups (470 ml) water

1 teaspoon kosher salt

½ teaspoon freshly ground black pepper

1. Drain and rinse the soaked beans in cold water.

2. Transfer the beans to a slow cooker, along with the carrots, celery, onions, mushrooms, tomatoes, garlic, tomato paste, and Italian seasoning. Stir to combine.

3. Add the broth and water, cover, and cook on HIGH for 3 to 4 hours, or until very tender.

4. Season with salt and pepper.

Serves 4

CASHEW CREAM:

½ cup (60 g) raw cashews

½ cup (120 ml) water

½ cup (6 g) cilantro leaves

Zest of 1 lime

3 tablespoons (45 ml) fresh lime juice

1 clove garlic, peeled

½ teaspoon garlic powder

½ teaspoon kosher salt

PEPPERS:

1 cup (235 ml) vegetable broth

½ cup (90 g) sprouted dry quinoa

2 tablespoons (30 ml) avocado oil

½ cup (71 g) finely chopped sweet onion

½ cup (71 g) finely chopped peeled carrots

½ cup (71 g) finely chopped celery

½ cup (1¼ oz [35 g]) finely chopped button mushrooms

1 can (14.5 ounces [411 g]) diced tomatoes, with their juice

1 teaspoon minced garlic

4 cups (2 oz [57 g]) baby spinach

½ teaspoon kosher salt

¼ teaspoon freshly ground black pepper

4 large red or yellow bell peppers

1. To make the cashew cream: Add cashews to a medium bowl and cover with boiling water. Soak for 1 hour, drain, and rinse.

2. Add the soaked cashews to a high-speed blender. Add the water, cilantro, lime zest and juice, garlic, garlic powder, and salt. Blend on high until smooth and creamy. Transfer to a bowl and set aside.

3. To make the peppers: Preheat the oven to 400°F (200°C, or gas mark 6).

4. In a small saucepan over medium heat, add the vegetable broth and quinoa. Bring to a boil, cover, reduce heat, and gently simmer for 10 to 12 minutes, until the quinoa is light and fluffy, all the broth is absorbed, and the kernels pop open. Turn off the heat and allow to sit for 5 minutes. Remove lid and fluff quinoa with a fork.

5. Meanwhile, in a large sauté pan over medium heat, add the avocado oil. Once hot, add the onions, carrots, celery, and mushrooms. Sauté, stirring occasionally, for 5 to 7 minutes, or until tender.

6. Stir in the tomatoes and garlic.

7. Add the spinach and cook, stirring occasionally, for 3 to 4 minutes, or until the spinach is wilted. Turn off the heat, add the quinoa, and stir to combine. Season with salt and pepper.

8. While the vegetables are cooking, prepare the peppers. Cut the peppers in half lengthwise. Remove and discard the seeds and membranes.

9. Fill the peppers with the quinoa-spinach mixture and place in a 3-quart (2.8 L) rectangular baking dish. Cover with a tight-fitting lid or foil.

10. Transfer to the oven and bake for 30 minutes. Uncover and cook an additional 5 minutes, or until the peppers are tender and the topping is browned and bubbly.

11. Remove from the oven and serve with the cashew cream.

QUINOA AND SPINACH–STUFFED PEPPERS WITH CASHEW CREAM

Quinoa is a high-protein seed and is so versatile. This stuffed pepper recipe is a delightful change to the meat-laden version that is more common. The cashew cream on top is a light and fresh topping that makes this pepper extra special. Soak the cashews first so you can prepare the peppers while they soak.

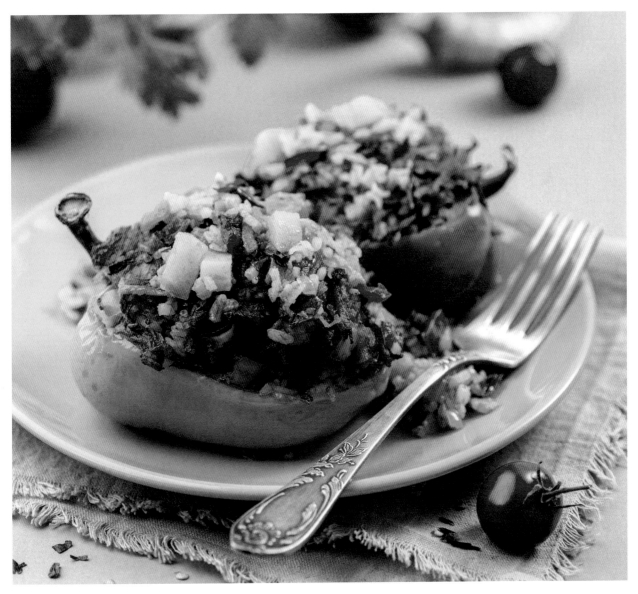

LAYERED VEGETABLE TACO SALAD IN A CRISPY BOWL

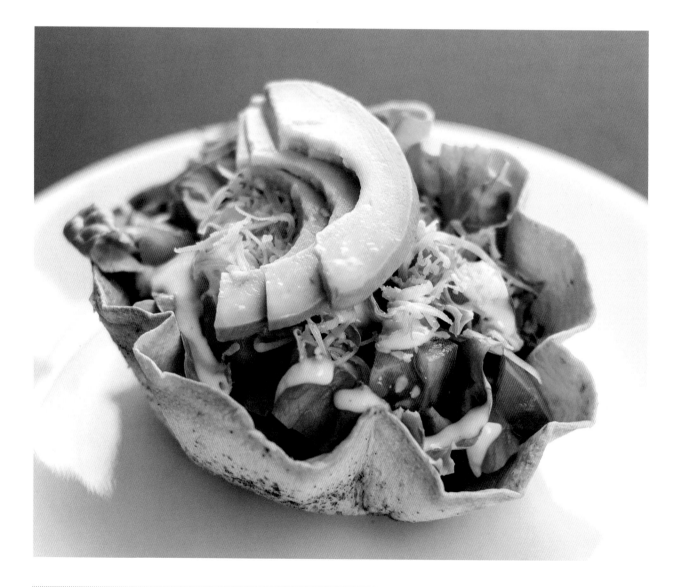

This taco salad is so delicious and filling and chock full of vegetables. The taco bowl is a simple baked tortilla shell that makes this salad a showstopper.

Serves 4

4 sprouted whole-grain tortillas (8 inch [20 cm])

1 can (15 ounces [425 g]) black beans, undrained

2 tablespoons (30 g) canned green chiles

½ teaspoon ground cumin

¼ teaspoon kosher salt

4 cups (80 g) chopped romaine

2 cups (304 g) frozen corn, thawed

1 pint (341 g) cherry tomatoes, halved

1 orange bell pepper, thinly sliced (about 1 cup)

¼ cup (28 g) grated hard cheese (optional)

2 ripe avocados, thinly sliced

1 cup (240 g) great-quality chunky salsa

¼ cup (3 g) cilantro, chopped

½ teaspoon kosher salt

1. Preheat the oven to 350˚F (180˚C, or gas mark 4). Turn over four oven-safe 4-inch (10-cm) ramekins or small bowls so the bottoms are facing up and spray lightly with cooking spray. Place on a baking sheet.

2. Set a tortilla on each ramekin, allowing the tortillas to fall over the ramekins to form a bowl.

3. Transfer the tortillas to the oven and bake for 12 to 15 minutes, or until lightly browned and crispy. Remove from the oven and allow to cool before removing from the ramekins.

4. Meanwhile, make the beans. In a small saucepan over low heat, combine the black beans with liquid, the green chiles, cumin, and salt. Heat until just simmering, then remove from heat.

5. To prepare the salads, arrange a tortilla bowl on each of 4 plates. Divide the beans between the bowls. Top with the romaine, corn, cherry tomatoes, peppers, and cheese (if desired).

6. Divide the sliced avocado between the 4 salads. Top with salsa and sprinkle with cilantro and salt. Serve immediately.

Picnics after church in Loma Linda are a place to be with community and gather around great food. Salads like this one are vegetable-forward, hearty dishes that showcase the fresh produce of California.

Serves 4

6 ounces (170 g) haricot verts or green beans

2 pounds (907 g) new potatoes

¼ cup (60 ml) extra-virgin olive oil

4 teaspoons (20 ml) fresh lemon juice

4 teaspoons (20 g) whole-grain mustard

½ cup (78 g) thinly sliced shallots

1 teaspoon chopped fresh thyme

1 teaspoon chopped fresh parsley

1 teaspoon chopped fresh basil

1 teaspoon chopped fresh dill

1 teaspoon kosher salt

1 can (15.5 ounces [439 g]) chickpeas, drained and rinsed

1. Bring a medium pot of salted water to a boil. Add the haricot verts and cook for 3 to 4 minutes, or until crisp tender. Remove from the boiling water with a slotted spoon and add to a bowl of ice water.

2. Add the potatoes to the same pot of boiling water. Reduce the heat to medium and simmer for 12 to 15 minutes, or until knife tender. Remove from the boiling water with a slotted spoon and allow to cool slightly. Once cool, cut the potatoes in half.

3. Meanwhile, in a large bowl, whisk together the olive oil, lemon juice, mustard, shallot, fresh herbs, and salt. Add in the (drained) haricot verts, potatoes, and chickpeas. Gently toss.

4. Serve warm or cold.

CHICKPEA, GREEN BEAN, AND NEW POTATO SALAD WITH HERB DRESSING

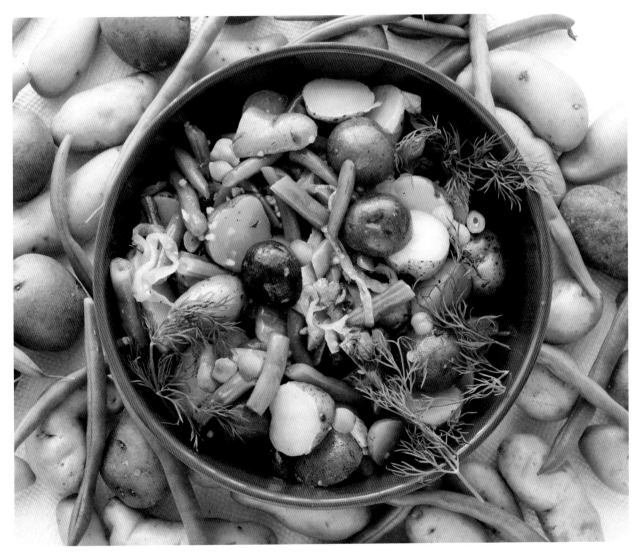

MEXICAN STUFFED SWEET POTATOES

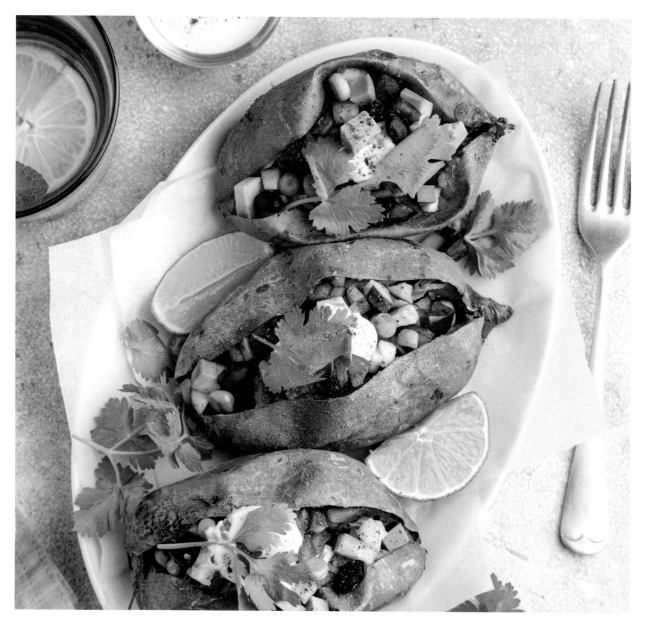

These stuffed potatoes are easily the perfect main dish or an incredible side dish. This recipe uses classic Mexican ingredients like tomato, cilantro, corn, and black beans. Stuffed into sweet potatoes and topped with guacamole and drizzled with vegan sour cream, you've got a winning dish.

Serves 4 as a main, 8 as a side

POTATOES:

4 medium sweet potatoes

1 tablespoon (15 ml) avocado oil

1 can (15 ounces [425 g]) black beans, drained and rinsed

1 cup (170 g) cherry tomatoes, quartered

½ cup (76 g) frozen corn, thawed

½ cup (6 g) fresh cilantro, chopped

¼ cup (36 g) finely chopped red onion

2 tablespoons (30 ml) fresh lime juice

2 teaspoons (10 ml) olive oil

1 clove garlic, minced

1 teaspoon kosher salt

GUACAMOLE:

1 ripe avocado

2 teaspoons (10 ml) fresh lime juice

½ teaspoon kosher salt

SOUR CREAM:

½ cup (114 g) plain coconut or almond yogurt, or regular plain yogurt

1 teaspoon lime zest

1 teaspoon fresh lime juice

¼ teaspoon kosher salt

1 lime, cut into 8 wedges, for garnish

1. To make the potatoes: Preheat the oven to 400°F (200°C, or gas mark 6). Line a baking sheet with parchment paper.

2. Using a fork, pierce holes in the potatoes and place on the prepared baking sheet. Drizzle with avocado oil. Transfer to the oven and bake for 45 minutes to 1 hour, or until they are knife tender.

3. Meanwhile, in a medium bowl, combine the black beans, tomatoes, corn, cilantro, red onion, lime juice, olive oil, garlic, and salt. Set aside.

4. To make the guacamole: In a small bowl, use a fork to mash together the flesh of the avocado with the lime juice and salt. Set aside. (If there's a lot of time left on the potatoes, cover the guacamole with a lid or plastic wrap.)

5. To make the sour cream: In another small bowl, combine the yogurt, lime zest and juice, and salt. Set aside.

6. To serve as a main dish, split the sweet potatoes lengthwise and divide the bean mixture among them. To serve as a side dish, cut the sweet potatoes in half then top the halves with the beans. Finish by dolloping the guacamole, drizzling with cream, and garnishing with a lime wedge for spritzing.

These simple 5–ingredient no–bake cookies are bursting with flavors and so chewy. Use certified gluten–free oats to make them gluten free. You can also switch up the nut butter you use, but I find almond butter makes the best cookies.

Makes 18

1 cup (250 g) natural creamy almond butter

½ cup (120 ml) pure maple syrup

1½ cups (220 g) sprouted rolled oats

½ cup (75 g) raisins

1 teaspoon ground cinnamon

1. Line a baking sheet with parchment paper and set aside.

2. In a small saucepan over low heat, add the almond butter and maple syrup. Whisk until well incorporated. Heat, stirring occasionally, until the mixture begins to bubble. Remove from heat.

3. In a large bowl, combine the oats, raisins, and cinnamon.

4. Pour the almond butter mixture over the dry ingredients and use a wooden spoon to combine.

5. Using a 2–tablespoon (30–ml) cookie scoop, scoop dough and drop onto the prepared baking sheet. Place scoops 2 inches (5 cm) apart.

6. Flatten cookies with a fork to desired thickness.

7. Transfer the baking sheet to the freezer and chill for 25 to 30 minutes.

8. Store in an airtight container in the refrigerator for up to 2 weeks.

NO-BAKE OATMEAL-RAISIN COOKIES

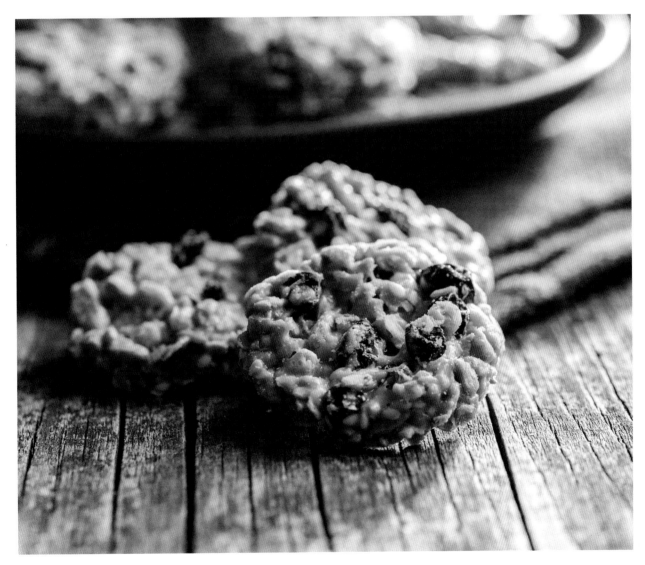

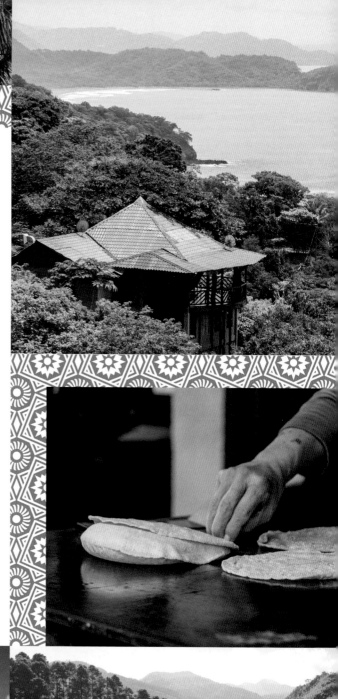

CHAPTER 4

NICOYA, COSTA RICA

This small rural community is on a gorgeous peninsula surrounded by lush mountains. What used to be volcanos is now dense green rainforest with ideal soil for farming. While it's a hub for tourism, it's also a place that thrives on preserving its traditional ways of life, a contrast of past and present. Nicoya is about four hours from San José, the capital of Costa Rica. This hard-working farming community is known for its smiles and willingness to help whenever necessary, living life by the motto *pura vida*, or "pure life." The roots of the Nicoyans are indigenous Chorotega, and their traditions enable them to live a relatively stress-free life. According to research, most Nicoyans live to at least the age of 90, and most live more than 100 years—many without age-related disease or disability. In fact, Nicoya has the highest number of centenarians in the world.

A Day in the Life

Starting the day at dawn is common in this farming region. A healthy breakfast is necessary for the hard work that comes throughout the day; rice and beans (*gallo pinto*), a homemade basket of corn tortillas, fresh fruit, and hot coffee is the norm. The men ride off on their horses to tend to the fields and use their machetes to clear rainforest, getting ready to cultivate the land for their crops; the women stay back and do the housework, milk the cows, feed the animals, and prepare the next meal.

Nicoyans eat nutritious food throughout the day, all grown on their own lands. Meat is eaten sometimes, but not often. The chemical free, naturally organic way of farming is a continuation of the traditional way things have been done for as long as these farmers can remember.

The tortilla has a very prominent place here in Nicoya, and it is eaten with almost every meal; in fact, corn (in some form) is one of the main components of everyday eating. Interestingly, the eating of maize or corn is what the locals attribute to their longevity. Some also say the traditional way of cooking their heirloom corn with wood ashes, called nixtamalization, is what makes the people of Nicoya rarely break a bone.

Another tradition is coyol, a drink that is native to Nicoya. Made from the sap of the coyol palm tree, it is said that this drink helps lengthen the lives of Nicoyans. It is used to combat anemia and diabetes, to regulate cholesterol and triglycerides, and to control high blood pressure. Naturally fermented with a coconut flavor, this drink comes in sweet, medium, and strong and is consumed throughout the day. The sweet variety is the fresh sap with little or no alcohol from the natural fermentation; the strong wine variety has the highest level of natural alcohol and a salty taste.

The traditional diet is not the only thing that has stayed the same; Nicoyans still love to walk from destination to destination and attribute their good physical and mental health to this. It also helps them maintain relationships within their communities. Being out in nature and appreciating all it has to offer is part of daily living. Rising with the sun, as well as the hard work, make the afternoon siesta necessary. Living with the natural rhythms of the sun means laying low when the heat is at its peak. Resting and regrouping is part of a natural and traditional cycle that makes up daily life here.

The biggest festivity of the year, *Las Fiestas Cívicas de Cobano*, takes place in mid–February and lasts for two weeks. The authentic and cheerful atmosphere of a Costa Rican fiesta is filled with customary food and music, proud horse riders, and bull riding. Cattle raising is a traditional lifestyle in Nicoya and the cowboys, or *sabaneros*, are well respected. The talent of these bull riders is revered and culminates in the National Championship.

As the day winds down in Nicoya, it ends much the same way it began, with good food, surrounded by family and those who have become family, community, and laughter. The sunset brings the end of the day and for most, bedtime. This way of life, from the outside at least, looks challenging and hard, but to the Nicoyan people it is the chosen way of life and a life well lived.

The Food of Nicoya

The Nicoya peninsula is where the people seem to elude heart disease, diabetes, and many forms of cancer, and this is attributed to their traditional cowboy lifestyle and way of eating. This community of hard-working people are known to eat the same thing almost every day for breakfast, lunch, and dinner. Meat and seafood make up only about 5 percent of the daily diet; the rest is dried beans, corn, squashes, yams, papaya and other tropical fruits, and white rice. Food grown by the people eating it, in the traditions of their people, served with love and intention, that's the Nicoyan way.

DRIED BEANS Black beans and pinto beans are the most-often-eaten legumes of Nicoya, but dried beans in general are a staple. They are rich in micronutrients such as potassium, magnesium, folate, iron, and zinc. An inexpensive form of protein, fiber, and iron, these amino acid–rich legumes are the building blocks that the body uses to heal and make new tissues such as bone, muscle, hair, skin, and blood.

CORN Corn is rich in dietary fiber, providing bulk to a mainly plant-based diet. It is also rich in the antioxidant vitamin C that helps protect cells from damage, helping prevent cancer and heart disease. The yellow variety is a good source of the carotenoids lutein and zeaxanthin, which are excellent for eye health. Nicoyans eat corn tortillas daily, freshly made by soaking dried corn in lime and water. This technique plays a major role in the absorption of vitamins and minerals; specifically, it aids in releasing the corn's niacin, which helps the body to absorb calcium, iron, and other valuable minerals.

YAMS AND SWEET POTATOES The yam is a fiber-rich tuber; it's a great source of potassium, magnesium, copper, and antioxidants. Yams have been linked to boosting brain health, reducing inflammation, and improving blood sugar control. They are rough and brown with a scaly skin, have white flesh, are long and cylindrical, and are dry and starchy. Sweet potatoes are a great source of fiber, vitamins, and minerals. They promote gut health by being a wonderful prebiotic, have cancer fighting properties, support healthy vision, enhance brain function, and help to support your immune system. The sweet potato is smooth with a thin orange skin, has orange, white, or purple flesh, is short and blocky in shape, and is moist and sweet in flavor.

SQUASHES Many varieties of squash are eaten daily in Nicoya. (In fact, the staples of beans, corn, and squash are called the three sisters; when grown together, they benefit each other in a variety of ways.) Squash has several health benefits including being beneficial for cardiovascular health, helping to maintain a healthy weight, improving eye health, reducing the risk of depression, and enhancing skin health.

CHAYOTE SQUASH The chayote squash, also known as mirliton, is a member of the gourd family. It has pale green flesh and is crisp when eaten raw and soft and creamy when cooked. Chayote is a great source of folate, with a whopping 40 percent of the recommended daily intake. Chayote also contains a compound that helps protect against the buildup of fat in the liver and helps the body to metabolize fats. It contains phytochemicals that help improve blood flow and reduce blood pressure levels. It is also rich in antioxidants like myricetin, which helps lower cholesterol levels, reduce inflammation, and protects against free radicals.

CILANTRO This amazing herb has been found to reduce the symptoms of cognitive diseases such as Alzheimer's and Parkinson's, reduce the number of seizure attacks, prevent nerve cell damage, reduce anxiety, help lower blood sugar, and, with its antimicrobial compounds, prevent foodborne illnesses. Cilantro is also a source of vitamins A, C, and K and contains folate, potassium, and manganese.

LIMES This fruit is high in antioxidants and vitamin C, both of which may help improve immunity, reduce the risk of heart disease, aid in iron absorption, prevent kidney stones, and even promote healthy skin. Limes are also a good source of magnesium and potassium.

CHAN SEEDS This tiny seed is native to Costa Rica and other parts of Central and South America; it resembles the chia seed and similarly boasts many health benefits. The chan seed is rich in protein and some essential amino acids, and it is packed with omega-3 and omega-6 fatty acids. These tiny seeds also contain potassium, calcium, fiber, zinc, iron, and vitamins A, B, C, and E. Most notably, they are high in magnesium, which has been shown to help manage stress, maintain blood pressure and blood sugar levels, aid in sleep regulation, and reduce cardiovascular risk factors.

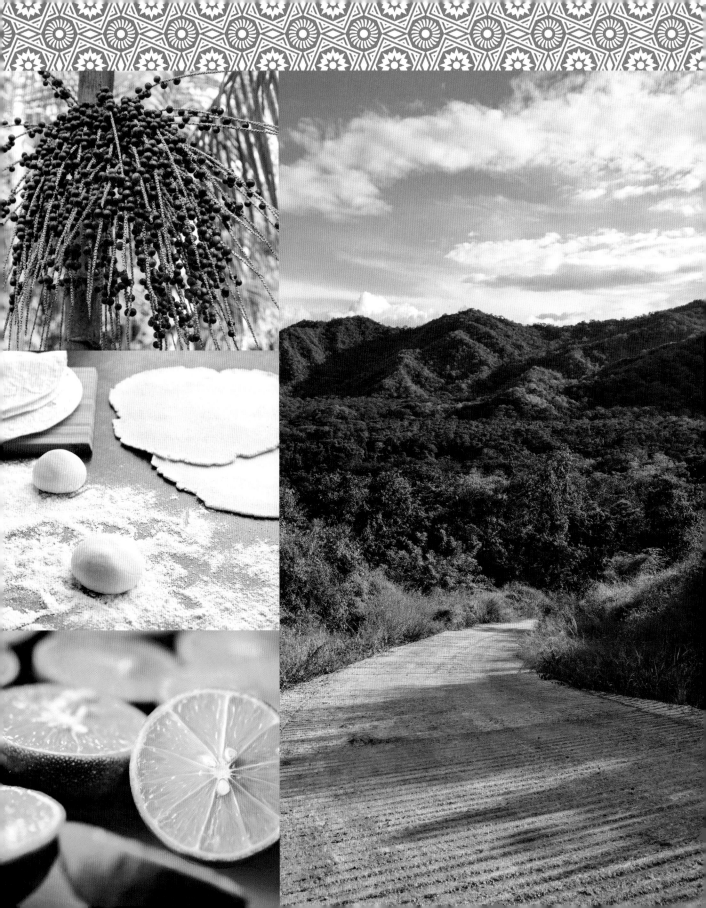

The Recipes of Nicoya

AÇAÍ SMOOTHIE BOWL WITH CHAN SEEDS

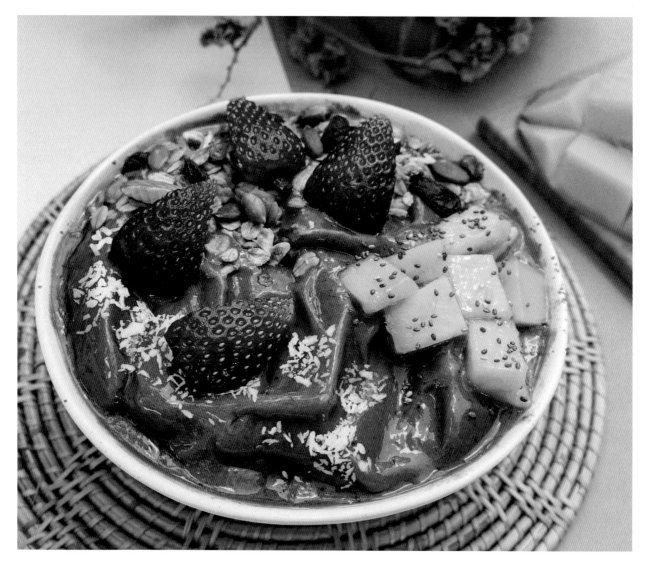

Smoothie bowls are a favorite of mine, and while not a traditional breakfast of Nicoya, the individual components are widely eaten there. The bowl has everything you need to start the day off right—protein, fiber, fat—and it's gorgeous! Feel free to play with the nuts and frozen fruits, and of course if you can't find chan seeds (check online), you may use chia instead.

Serves 2

2 peeled and sliced frozen bananas

2 packets (200 g) frozen açaí puree

1 cup (150 g) frozen strawberries

1 cup (150 g) frozen blueberries

1½ cups (350 ml) oat or almond milk

½ cup (128 g) plain or almond milk Greek yogurt

1 cup (170 g) sliced or diced fresh mango

½ cup (40 g) unsweetened toasted coconut flakes

½ cup (60 g) chopped toasted mixed nuts (almonds, hazelnuts, macadamia)

¼ cup (52 g) chan or chia seeds

1. Place the bananas, açaí, strawberries, blueberries, milk, and yogurt in a high-powered blender. Puree on medium, tapping down with a tamper in between to make sure the fruit is getting blended. Puree until smooth.

2. Divide the smoothie between 2 bowls. Top with the mango, coconut flakes, nuts, and chan seeds. Enjoy immediately.

This hash is so easy and so tasty! The potatoes take a little bit of time to become browned and crispy, so plan accordingly. You may use all sweet potatoes or all russet potatoes if that's what you have. The combination of russet potatoes, sweet potatoes, corn, and tomatoes is perfect on its own, but feel free to top it with an egg if you wish.

Serves 4

2 medium russet potatoes, peeled and cut into ½-inch pieces (about 1½ cups)

1 medium sweet potato, peeled and cut into ½-inch pieces (about 1½ cups)

2 cups (470 ml) water

1 tablespoon (15 ml) white wine vinegar

1 teaspoon kosher salt, divided

⅓ cup (80 ml) olive oil

1½ cups (228 g) fresh corn kernels

1 cup (170 g) cherry tomatoes, halved

½ teaspoon freshly ground black pepper

¼ cup (3 g) fresh cilantro, chopped

1. Heat a 12-inch (30 cm) cast iron skillet over medium heat. Add both types of potatoes in a single layer, the water, vinegar, and ½ teaspoon salt.

2. Bring the mixture to a simmer, reduce the heat to medium-low and allow the potatoes to cook for about 20 minutes, stirring once, or until the potatoes are tender and the water has evaporated.

3. Increase the heat to medium-high, add the olive oil, and allow to cook without stirring for 7 to 10 minutes, or until the potatoes are browned and crispy on the bottom. Continue to cook an additional 5 to 7 minutes, stirring frequently, until all the potatoes are browned and crispy.

4. Add the corn, tomatoes, remaining ½ teaspoon salt, and black pepper. Stir to combine and cook for 2 to 3 minutes, or until the tomatoes and corn are warmed through.

5. Transfer to a serving plate and sprinkle with cilantro.

POTATO, SWEET POTATO, CORN, AND TOMATO HASH

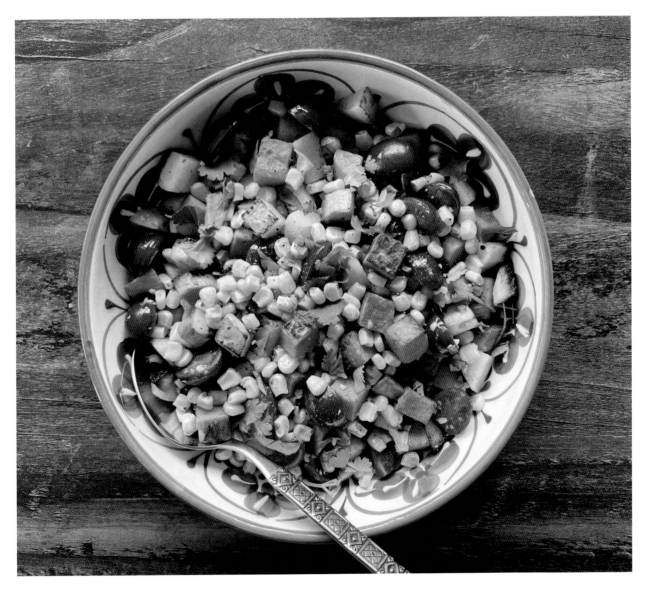

BLACK BEAN, LIME, AND TOMATO SOUP

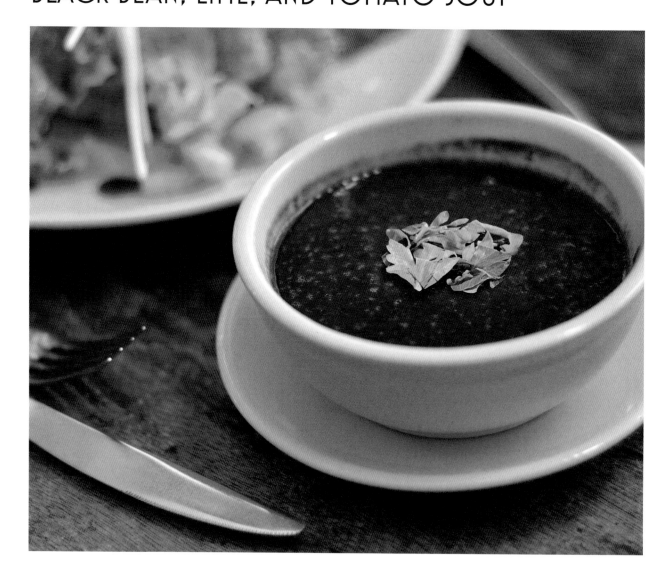

This combination of lime, tomato, and black beans makes for an unforgettable soup. Canned black beans make it super quick and easy. Serve with the Homemade Tortillas on page 94 for a simple and hearty meal.

Serves 6

1 tablespoon (15 ml) avocado oil

1 cup (142 g) diced white onion

½ cup (71 g) peeled and diced carrot

4 cloves garlic, minced

2 teaspoons (5 g) ground cumin

2 cans (15 ounces [425 g]) black beans, undrained

2 cups (750 g) chopped Roma tomatoes

1 quart (946 ml) vegetable broth

2 tablespoons (4 g) lime zest

2 tablespoons (30 ml) fresh lime juice

1 tablespoon (15 ml) hot sauce

½ teaspoon kosher salt

¼ cup (3 g) fresh cilantro, chopped

1. In a large stock pot over medium heat, add the oil. Once hot, add the onions and carrots and sauté, stirring frequently, for 5 to 8 minutes, or until the onions are lightly browned and tender.

2. Add the garlic and cumin and stir for 30 seconds.

3. Stir in the black beans with liquid, tomatoes, and broth. Bring to a boil. Reduce heat to medium low and simmer for 20 minutes, stirring occasionally.

4. Transfer half of the soup to a blender, add the lime zest and juice, hot sauce, and salt. Puree until smooth and creamy.

5. Transfer back to the stock pot and stir to combine the pureed and unpureed soup. Ladle into bowls and top with fresh cilantro.

This creamy butternut squash soup is so complex in flavor and simple in ingredients, it will quickly become a favorite!

Serves 6

4 pounds (1.8 kg) butternut squash

1 medium onion

3 tablespoons (45 ml) avocado oil, divided

10 cloves garlic, peeled

1 tablespoon (6 g) grated fresh ginger

1 teaspoon ground cumin

1 teaspoon ground cinnamon

¼ teaspoon ground nutmeg

6 cups (1.4 L) vegetable broth

1 bay leaf

1 teaspoon kosher salt

½ teaspoon freshly cracked black pepper

½ cup (60 g) toasted and salted pepitas

1. Preheat the oven to 400°F (200°C, or gas mark 6). Line a baking sheet with parchment paper and set aside.

2. Cut the squash in half lengthwise, scoop out the seeds and membranes and transfer, cut side down, to the prepared baking sheet.

3. Cut the onion in half, peel, and add the halves, cut side down, to the baking sheet. Drizzle the squash and onion with 1 tablespoon (15 ml) of the avocado oil and transfer to the oven.

4. Bake for 40 to 50 minutes, or until the squash is tender and the onions are caramelized. Allow to cool for a few minutes. Once cool enough to touch, scoop out the squash flesh and discard the skin.

5. Add the remaining 2 tablespoons (30 ml) of oil to a large pot set over medium heat. Add the squash, roasted onions, garlic, ginger, cumin, cinnamon, and nutmeg. Stir to coat in all the spices.

6. Add the vegetable broth, bay leaf, salt, and pepper and bring to a boil over medium-high heat.

7. Reduce the heat to low and simmer for 7 to 10 minutes, or until all the flavors have a chance to meld.

8. Remove from heat, remove the bay leaf, and pour the soup, in batches, into a high-powered blender. Blend until smooth and creamy.

9. Pour into bowls and garnish with the toasted pepitas.

ROASTED BUTTERNUT SQUASH SOUP WITH PEPITAS

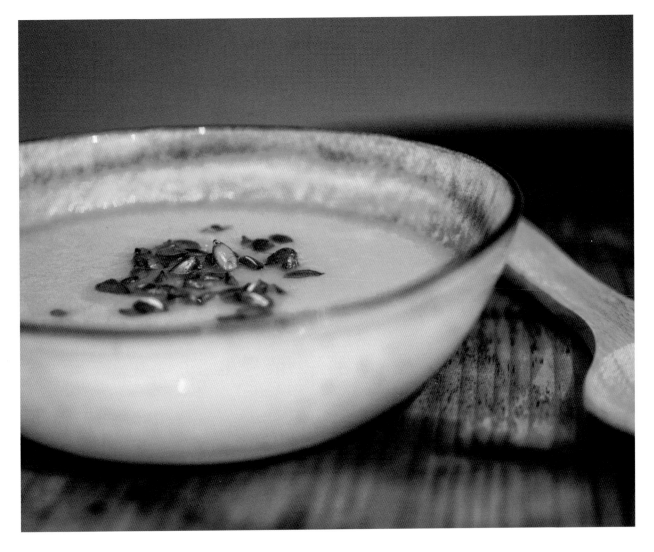

CORN, PINTO BEAN, AND PEPPER–STUFFED CHAYOTE

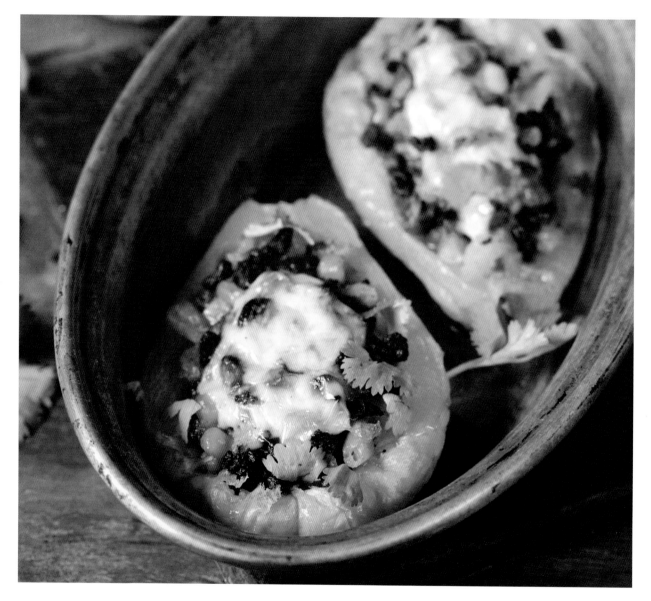

This mild-flavored chayote squash, also known as mirliton, is stuffed with "the three sisters"; this combination of corn, beans, and squash is a traditional one in Nicoyan cuisine. The three crops are planted together to support and nourish one another. If you can't find chayote, try this dish with zucchini or crookneck squash instead.

Serves 6

3 chayote squash

2 tablespoons (30 ml) avocado oil

1 cup (142 g) diced red onion

½ cup (57 g) chopped red bell pepper

½ cup (57 g) chopped yellow bell pepper

2 cloves garlic, minced

1 teaspoon ground cumin

1 teaspoon chili powder

1 teaspoon dried oregano

1 can (15 ounces [425 g]) pinto beans, undrained

1 cup (152 g) fresh corn kernels

¼ cup (28 g) grated hard cheese (optional)

¼ cup (3 g) cilantro, chopped

1. Bring a large pot of salted water to a boil over medium-high heat.

2. Slice the chayote in half lengthwise. Add halved squash to the boiling water and boil for 30 minutes. Drain.

3. Meanwhile, preheat the oven to 375°F (190°C, or gas mark 5). Line a baking sheet with parchment paper.

4. When the squash is cool enough to handle, scoop out the seeds and discard. Scoop out the flesh and reserve, leaving a 1-inch boat border. Arrange the 6 shells cut side up on the prepared baking sheet. Set aside.

5. In a large sauté pan over medium heat, add the avocado oil. Once hot, add the red onion, bell peppers, and garlic. Sauté, stirring occasionally, for 5 to 7 minutes, or until lightly browned and tender.

6. Stir in the cumin, chili powder, and oregano and stir for 30 seconds, or until fragrant.

7. Add the reserved chayote, pinto beans with liquid, and corn. Cook for 5 minutes, or until the corn is tender and everything is well combined. Remove from heat.

8. Divide the filling mixture among the 6 shells.

9. Transfer to the oven and bake for 25 to 30 minutes, or until lightly browned and hot. Top with grated cheese, if desired, and pop back into the oven until melted.

10. Serve topped with chopped cilantro.

Beans and rice are a pairing that makes up breakfast, lunch, and dinner in Nicoya. This tomato rice is flavorful and a perfect side dish to a pot of beans and Homemade Tortillas (page 94).

Serves 8

2 tablespoons (30 ml) avocado oil

2 cups (396 g) long grain rice

1 quart (946 ml) vegetable or chicken broth

1 cup (250 g) canned tomato sauce

6 cilantro stems

1 clove garlic, minced

2 teaspoons (11 g) kosher salt, divided

½ teaspoon ground cumin

4 ripe avocados

Zest of 1 lime

2 tablespoons (30 ml) fresh lime juice

1. Heat the oil in a large heavy-bottomed pan over medium heat.

2. Add the rice and cook, stirring frequently, for 3 to 5 minutes, or until lightly browned.

3. Add the broth, tomato sauce, cilantro stems, garlic, 1 teaspoon salt, and cumin, and bring to a boil. Reduce the heat to low, cover, and cook for 20 minutes. Turn off the heat and allow to sit, covered, for 5 minutes.

4. White the rice is cooking, grill the avocados. Preheat a grill pan over high heat.

5. Slice the avocados in half lengthwise and remove the pits. Season with the remaining 1 teaspoon salt.

6. Grill, flesh side down, for 2 to 4 minutes, or until good grill marks form.

7. Remove from heat, scoop out the flesh with a spoon, and thinly slice.

8. To serve, divide the tomato rice among bowls, top with avocado, lime zest, and lime juice.

TOMATO RICE WITH
GRILLED AVOCADO AND LIME

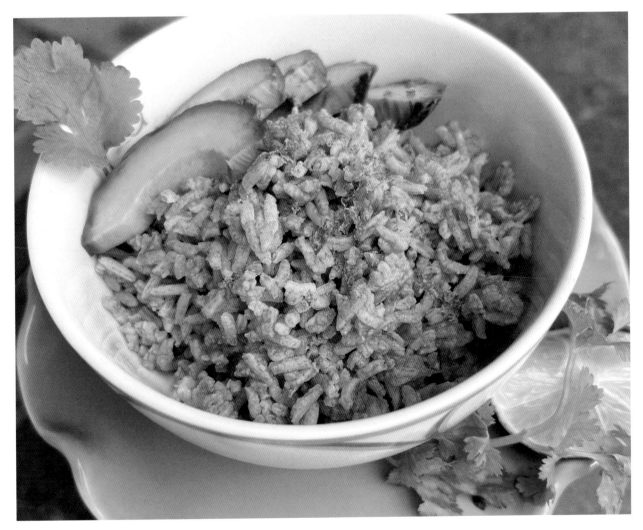

HOMEMADE TORTILLAS

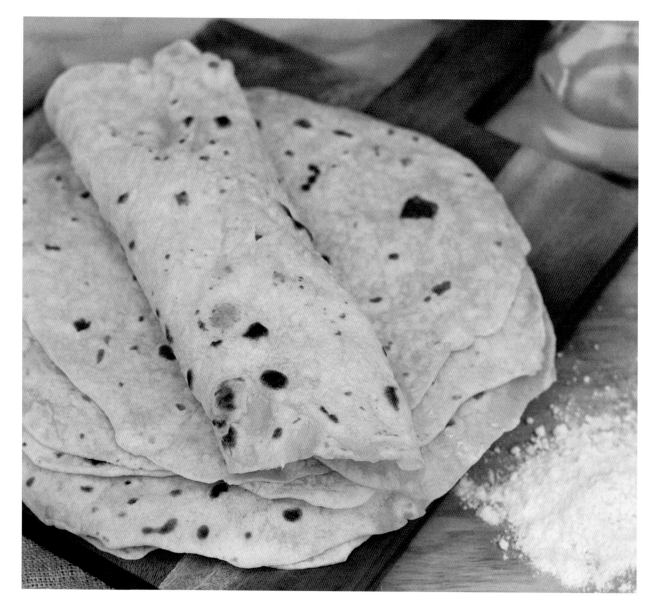

Homemade tortillas are a staple of Nicoyan life. These are not a replica of the ones you will find made there, but rather a substitute (and better than the store-bought ones you would find here). The tradition and love that goes into the Nicoyan-made tortillas requires lime water and a special dried corn that is stone ground daily. The ones we will be making are delicious and wonderful in their own right! Masa harina is a maize dough that comes from ground nixtamalized corn. It is used for making tortillas, tamale dough, gorditas, pupusas, and many other dishes. It is easily found in the baking section of most grocery stores or in specialty Hispanic markets.

Makes 12

2 cups (186 g) masa harina

½ teaspoon kosher salt

1½ cups (350 ml) warm water, divided

1. In a large bowl, mix the masa harina and salt.

2. Add 1 cup (235 ml) of the water and mix. The dough will look crumbly.

3. Adding 1 tablespoon (15 ml) at a time, add more water until the mixture forms a soft dough that holds together.

4. Separate the dough into golf ball–size pieces, and roll each one into a ball.

5. Cut two pieces of parchment paper or waxed paper, about 6 inches long each. Place one on the bottom and one on the top of a ball of dough. Place a large heavy skillet, or something equally heavy, on top of the dough and flatten. Remove the paper and set aside the tortilla, covering with a clean, damp kitchen towel. Repeat with the remaining dough until all the tortillas are made.

6. To cook, heat a large skillet over medium-high heat. Once hot, add the tortillas one at a time and cook for 1 minute on each side, or until charred spots form and they puff up. Keep them warm while you cook the remaining dough.

7. Serve by themselves or with your favorite toppings.

This refreshing fruit drink, literally "cool water," is made by blending ripe fruit with water and lime. Here, we've added chan seeds, which makes this not only more nutritious, but also more filling. If you cannot find them, feel free to substitute chia seeds. I love this as a dessert beverage, but also as a simple midday pick me up.

Serves 4

4 cups (946 ml) filtered water

1½ cups (204 g) fresh pineapple chunks

¼ cup (60 ml) fresh lime juice

3 tablespoons (39 g) chan or chia seeds

1. Add the water, pineapple, lime juice, and chan seeds to a high-speed blender. Puree on high until smooth and creamy.

2. Transfer the mixture to the refrigerator and allow to chill for 1 hour.

3. To serve, pour into glasses as is or pour over ice.

CHAN SEED–PINEAPPLE AGUA FRESCA

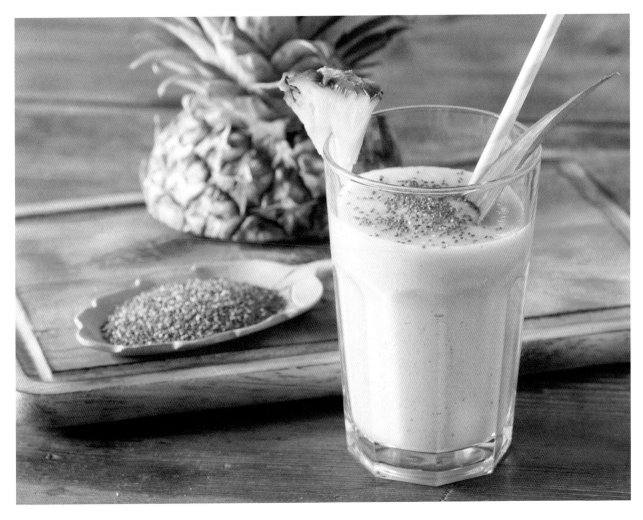

PINTO BEAN SALAD

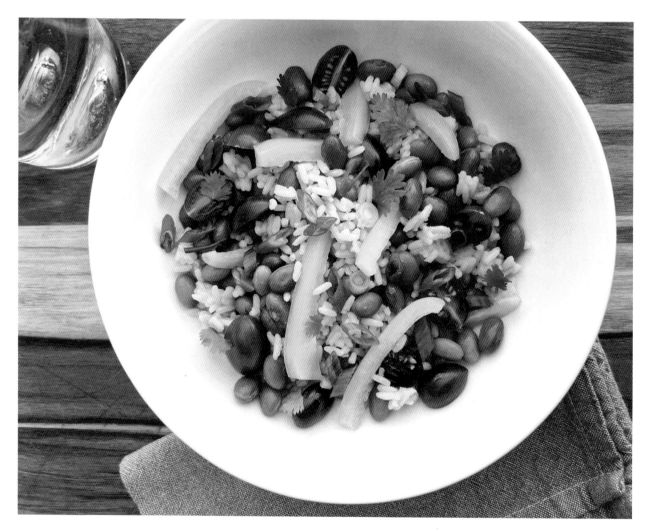

This simple salad is made incredible by the freshest of ingredients. Make sure you use tomatoes that are at their peak. The rest can be made quickly, especially if you are using leftover beans and rice. I am using canned beans here for ease of preparation, but use cooked dried beans if you wish.

Serves 6

2 cups (470 ml) water

1 cup (198 g) long grain rice

½ teaspoon kosher salt

1 can (15 ounces [425 g]) pinto beans, drained and rinsed

⅓ cup (80 ml) extra-virgin olive oil

2 tablespoons (30 ml) red wine vinegar

1 teaspoon minced garlic

1 pint (341 g) grape tomatoes, halved lengthwise

1 yellow bell pepper, thinly sliced (about 1 cup)

½ cup (32 g) chopped scallions

½ cup (6 g) cilantro leaves

1. In a medium saucepan, add the water, rice, and salt, and bring to a boil over medium–high heat. Reduce the heat to low, cover, and simmer for 15 minutes. Turn off the heat and allow to sit for 5 minutes. Uncover, fluff with a fork, and transfer to a large bowl. Allow to cool for 10 more minutes.

2. Once the rice has cooled, add the pinto beans, olive oil, red wine vinegar, and garlic. Toss to coat.

3. Add the tomatoes, bell pepper, scallions, and cilantro leaves. Gently toss and serve.

This shake, also called horchata, originated in southern Spain, but you can find versions of it all over the Americas, from Mexico to Ecuador. While the ingredients are simple, soaking it for 8 to 12 hours is necessary for the creamy consistency. Light and refreshing, this "sweetened rice milk" is a treat when it's hot out.

Serves 4

1 cup (198 g) long grain white rice

½ cup (43 g) sliced almonds

2 cinnamon sticks

3 cups (700 ml) water

½ cup (107 g) sugar

1 teaspoon vanilla extract

2 cups (470 ml) almond milk

1. In a high-speed blender, add the raw rice, almonds, and cinnamon sticks. Blend on high for 1 minute, or until finely pulverized, stopping occasionally and shaking if it sticks to the bottom.

2. Add in the water, sugar, and vanilla and blend an additional 30 seconds.

3. Add in the almond milk and blend until incorporated.

4. Transfer to a pitcher, cover, and refrigerate for 8 to 12 hours.

5. When ready to serve, strain the mixture through a fine-mesh strainer and serve over ice.

RICE SHAKE WITH VANILLA AND CINNAMON

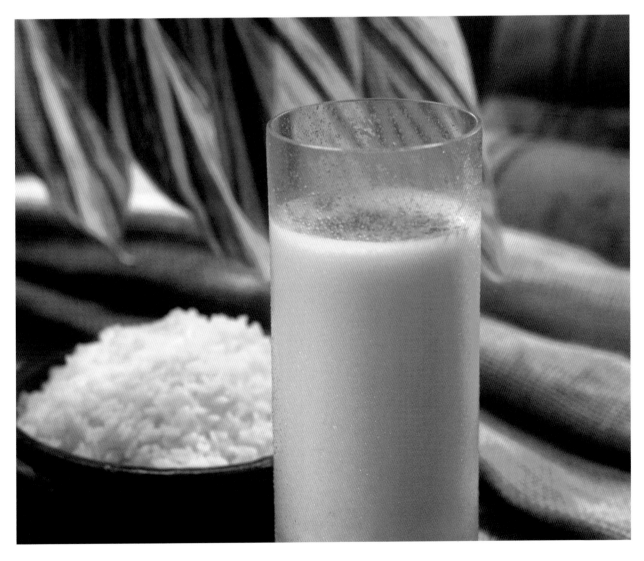

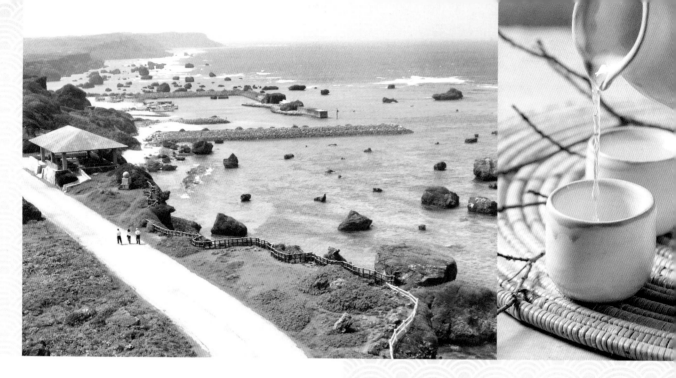

CHAPTER 5

OKINAWA, JAPAN

Off the coast of the southernmost tip of Japan lies Okinawa, a series of small islands that are lumped into three main groups. The main large one is the urban cultural center, also the capital Naha. These islands have a subtropical climate, turquoise waters, and exquisite sandy beaches. The history of Okinawa stretches back thousands of years to the Minatogawa people. In 2015, a study was done of centenarians in Okinawa and found that when compared to Japan as a whole, Okinawans had almost double the number of centenarians per 100,000 people, and women accounted for about 88 percent of them.

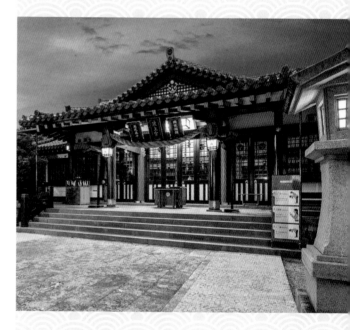

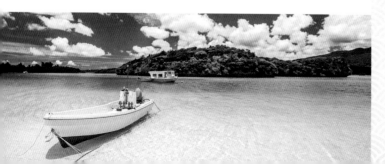

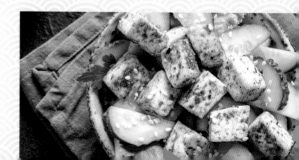

A Day in the Life

Sunrise starts the day in Okinawa, with light breaking through the clouds over the exquisite turquoise waters of this beautiful island. The day begins with prayers to ancestors, a ritual that is practiced to give thanks to the people who came before, honoring the spirits and allowing them to guide Okinawans through their lives. Prayers hold such an important part of the Okinawan lifestyle that they are the focus of annual events. These events are held according to the lunar calendar and range from welcoming ancestors, to wishing for a bountiful harvest and plentiful fishing, to praying for appreciation.

After prayers, a traditional breakfast of tofu miso soup and green or jasmine tea is had. This light breakfast may seem like lunch or dinner, but in Okinawa there isn't much variation between the meals. Walks along the white sand beaches, looking out at the surf, tend to follow breakfast, a walking meditation if you will. Afterward, time is spent in the garden, as almost all older Okinawans have a vegetable garden. This garden is just one more way they take care of themselves and each other, providing what they need to nourish their bodies with their own hands. After a little hard work in the garden, many still work the fields. In fact, it is not uncommon for Okinawans to still be doing manual labor at the age of 100!

A light lunch is often a time to meet with friends, children, grandchildren, or great-grandchildren; Okinawans prize their family and tend to spend some time each day together. Family, laughter, and gossip while eating a lunch of bitter melon, tofu, kelp, and whole grains such as millet, wheat, rice, and noodles, along with another cup of tea is standard here. These light meals employ what is referred to as *hara hachi bu*, which means to eat until you are 80 percent full; Okinawans attribute their longevity to this mindset. Lunch is typically followed by an afternoon nap, resting up from all the manual labor the morning held and sleeping during the warmest part of the afternoon.

After a nap, there's a meeting with one's *moai*, or friends who share one's common purpose in life. This group, which each person chooses for themselves, meets to address their social, financial, and personal needs. A little sake might be had during this time as well. This style of social therapy is made light with laughter, gossip, and a mutual desire to see each other thrive.

The sun is now setting over Okinawa, which means a time of reflection and dinner, a light meal of garden-grown vegetables, fermented tofu, and a cup of specialty mugwort sake (a sake steeped with mugwort that aids in digestion and treats anxiety). This life of fulfillment in one's surroundings, spent with those you love most, having your needs met by family and friends, and thanking ancestors for all the knowledge they have imparted, is a simple one. A life spent in the moment, being present with the earth and the body you are given. This island is known for fresh air, sunshine, and outdoor activities. The day closes with the setting sun.

The Food of Okinawa

The food of Okinawa was and is influenced by its long history of trade with China and Southeast Asia. The diet of these healthy and long-living people consists mainly of plants, with up to two servings of tofu daily; they eat very little meat and seafood, even though they live on an island. The nutrient-dense and unique foods that stand out in this cuisine are nutritional powerhouses.

JAPANESE PURPLE SWEET POTATO These beautiful tubers are loaded with vitamins, minerals, and antioxidants. Rich in anthocyanins, which give these tubers their brilliant color, they help reduce blood pressure and protect against inflammation, type 2 diabetes, and certain cancers. They are also a great source of vitamin C, potassium, and phytonutrients. These complex carbohydrates also offer up an amazing prebiotic, giving gut health a major boost. You may not be able to find the exact Okinawan purple sweet potato, or *beni imo*, where you live, but there are many purple varietals available that you can use as a substitute.

SHIITAKE MUSHROOMS These rich and savory mushrooms were used in ancient Asia as aphrodisiacs and as promoters of youthfulness and virility. They have cancer-fighting compounds, boost immunity, and support heart health. Additionally, they have polysaccharides, terpenoids, sterols, and lipids, all of which are great for the immune system, lowering cholesterol, controlling diabetes, and treating eczema.

BLACK TEA Japanese black tea contains a moderate amount of caffeine, which is great for just a little boost of energy. A compound called l-theanine is a component of black tea and helps reduce stress. This antioxidant-rich tea has also been shown to improve focus, mental clarity, and heart and gut health, as well as lower LDL or "bad" cholesterol, blood pressure, and blood sugar levels.

BITTER MELON This member of the gourd family, called *goya* in Japanese, is a very interesting vegetable indeed. Its flavor is bitter always, yet can be tamed when salted, sautéed, curried, or otherwise camouflaged with pungent spices. It has a watery texture like a cucumber and a crunchy outside like a green bell pepper. Sounds strange, yes, but its health benefits are incredible. This melon is a good source of fiber, vitamin C, folate, and vitamin A.

TOFU Tofu is not only a complete protein, it is also a nutrient powerhouse. This product of the soybean contains several anti-inflammatory and antioxidant phytochemicals. It is also a good source of fiber, potassium, magnesium, iron, copper, and manganese. Tofu is a blank canvas, absorbing flavors to make it a versatile star on any plate.

KOMBU This dried seaweed is traditionally used to flavor stocks and reduce the gas producing component in beans. Easily found in the international section of your grocery store or your local Asian market, there are many varieties; Hidaka is my personal favorite. Kombu has an incredible iodine content, which is essential for thyroid function, and it is known for reducing blood cholesterol and high blood pressure. It is high in iron, which helps distribute oxygen to cells, and is also a good source of calcium, vitamin A, and vitamin C.

MISO Miso translates to "fermented beans" in Japanese. The many varieties and colors of miso are attributed to the length of fermentation time, making it sweet and mild to salty and rich. This fermented paste is a probiotic that aids in gut health. The gut-brain connection is a well-studied one, and the findings are great in the gut's ability to help lower anxiety and depression while increasing immune function. The immune system has been front and center these past few years, and including pre- and probiotics in our diets is an easy and essential way to help the body maintain a healthy gut biome. Miso is found in the refrigerated section of most grocery stores.

KOKUTO SUGAR Okinawan black/brown sugar or kokuto sugar is a sugar like no other. (It's called by either color.) This sugar is cooked slowly from sugar cane grown on the islands, without adding or taking anything away from it. It has a rich, complex flavor that is the secret to many Japanese sweets and snacks. Its medicinal properties are also unmatched compared to other sugars. Kokuto is high in potassium, calcium, and iron—it contains even more iron than spinach. Kokuto sugar might be a little trickier to find than most ingredients. A well-stocked Asian market might have it, but the easiest place to find kokuto is online. If you cannot find it, a great substitute is coconut sugar, dark muscovado sugar, or even date sugar.

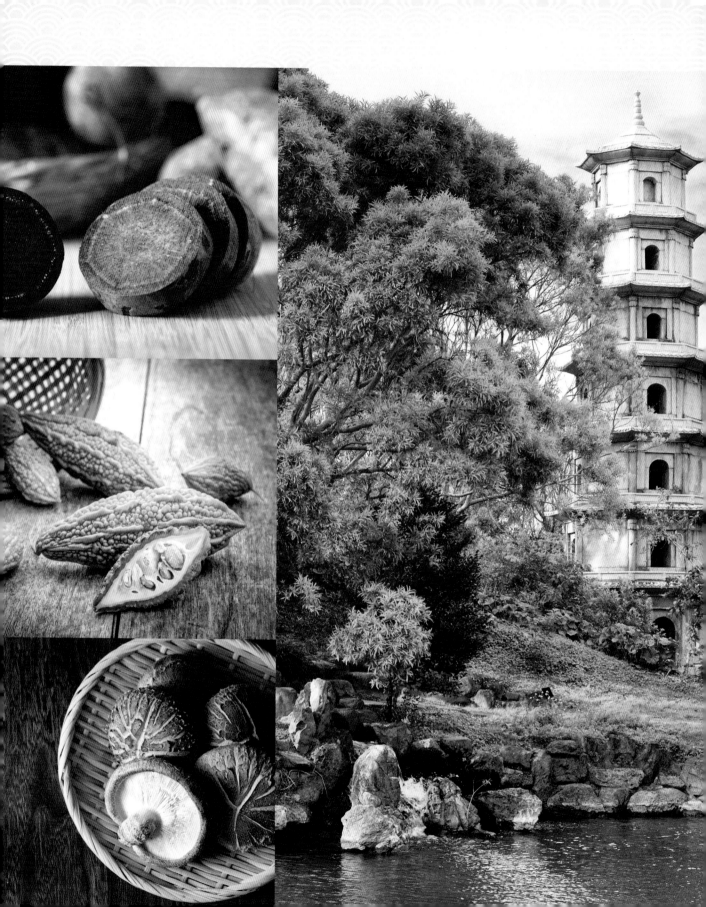

The Recipes of Okinawa

PURPLE SWEET POTATO, TOFU, AND SPINACH HASH

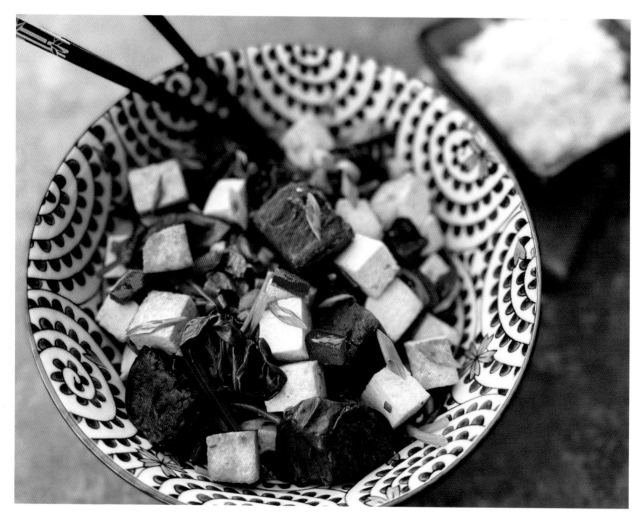

Hash is such a simple delicious breakfast. This may not be an authentic Okinawan dish, but it utilizes many of the ingredients that make up a typical Okinawan breakfast. Top it with a poached or fried egg if you wish, or serve with rice.

Serves 4

2 tablespoons avocado oil, divided

1 medium Okinawan purple sweet potato, cut into 1-inch cubes (about 2 cups)

¼ cup (60 ml) water

16 ounces (454 g) extra-firm or super-firm tofu, cut into ½-inch cubes

½ cup (71 g) chopped red onion

½ cup (71 g) chopped red bell pepper

2 cloves garlic, minced

5- or 6-ounce package (142 to 170 g) baby spinach

¼ cup (16 g) chopped scallions

½ teaspoon sea salt

½ teaspoon freshly ground black pepper

1 teaspoon tamari

1. In a large nonstick sauté pan over medium heat, add 1 tablespoon (15 ml) of the oil.

2. Add the sweet potato and water, cover, and cook for 8 to 10 minutes, or until the potatoes start to become tender crisp, and brown.

3. Remove the lid and sauté for 7 to 10 minutes longer. The water will evaporate, the yams will become more crisp and tender. Remove from the pan and set aside, keeping warm.

4. Heat the remaining 1 tablespoon (15 ml) avocado oil in the pan over medium heat. Add the tofu, onions, bell peppers, and garlic. Cook, stirring occasionally, for 8 to 10 minutes, or until the peppers and onions are tender. Add the potatoes back in, stirring to combine.

5. Add in the spinach and scallions, and season with salt and pepper. Stir for 1 to 2 minutes, or until the spinach is wilted. Stir in the tamari and serve.

Smoothies are such a simple, filling, and well-rounded breakfast. Here, the hemp seeds, rich in both omega-3 and omega-6 fatty acids, are an excellent addition with their heart-healthy compounds. The purple sweet potato contributes its own special and extra-nutritious kick, while the lemon juice adds a unique brightness.

Serves 2

1 cup (227 g) roasted purple sweet potato (skin removed)

12 strawberries

1 large peeled and sliced frozen banana

2 cups (470 ml) oat or soy milk

½ cup (120 ml) fresh lemon juice

½ teaspoon ground cinnamon

¼ teaspoon ground ginger

¼ teaspoon ground nutmeg

2 tablespoons (10 g) toasted coconut flakes

1 tablespoon (13 g) hemp seeds

1. Place the sweet potato, strawberries, banana, milk, lemon juice, and spices into a high-powered blender. Blend on high until smooth and creamy.

2. Pour into 2 glasses and top with the toasted coconut flakes and hemp seeds.

PURPLE SWEET POTATO–STRAWBERRY SMOOTHIE

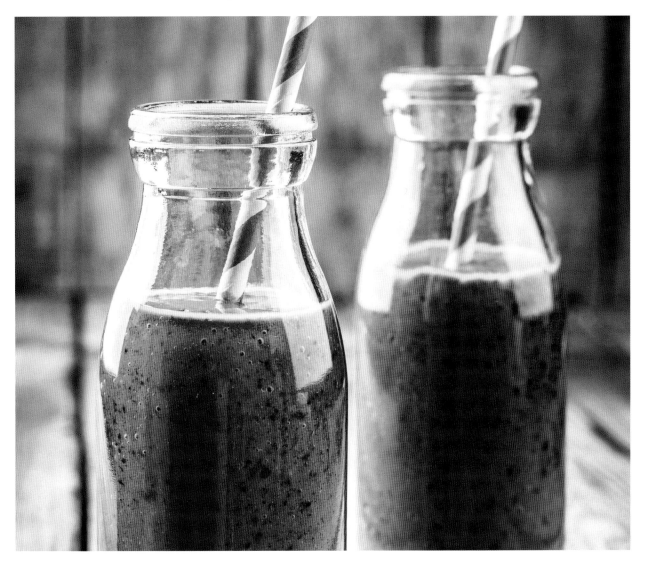

CHAMPURU (OKINAWAN TOFU AND VEGETABLES)

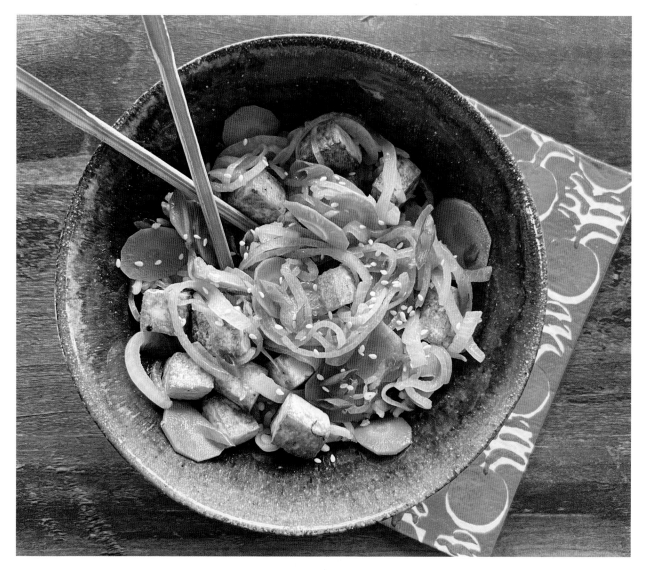

This is a spin on a traditional Okinawan dinner. The combination of tofu and veggies is called champuru, and it is the official representative dish of Okinawa. Oftentimes, fish or pork belly will be added. For a full meal, serve alongside a bowl of steamed sticky rice and miso soup. Have all vegetables cut and prepared before you start, as this dish comes together quickly.

Note: To press tofu, wrap in a clean, dry kitchen towel, set in a plate, cover with another plate or sheet pan, and place something heavy on top, like two large soup cans. Allow to sit for 30 minutes.

Serves 4

16 ounces (454 g) firm tofu, pressed then cut into ½-inch cubes (see Note)

2 tablespoons (30 ml) avocado oil

2 cups (284 g) thinly sliced yellow onion

1 cup (142 g) thinly sliced peeled carrots

1 tablespoon (15 ml) toasted sesame oil

2 tablespoons (30 ml) tamari

1 bunch scallions, white and green parts cut into 1-inch pieces (about 1 cup)

2 tablespoons (18 g) toasted sesame seeds

1. While the tofu is pressing, prepare the vegetables.

2. Place a wok or large sauté pan over medium-high heat, and add the avocado oil.

3. Add the onion and carrots and sauté for 4 to 5 minutes, or until the vegetables have some caramelization and are crisp tender. Remove from the pan.

4. Add the sesame oil to the pan and return to medium heat. Add the tofu and sauté for 4 to 5 minutes.

5. Add the tamari, carrots, onion, and scallions. Stir fry for 1 minute.

6. Remove from heat. Sprinkle with sesame seeds.

Goya champuru is the most well-known dish of Okinawa. Bitter melon, tofu, egg, and pork belly make up the original dish. Feel free to add crispy pork belly if you wish. You may swap the shiitake broth for dashi (see page 119) to make the dish even more authentic. Koregusu is a specialty ingredient made in Okinawa from Shima Togarashi chili peppers, infused into a traditional Okinawan high-proof spirit called awamori. It is quite spicy! If you can't find it in a specialty Asian market, feel free to substitute sriracha.

Note: To press tofu, wrap in a clean, dry kitchen towel, set in a plate, cover with another plate or sheet pan, and place something heavy on top, like two large soup cans. Allow to sit for 30 minutes.

Serves 4

16 ounces (454 g) extra-firm tofu, pressed (see Note)

1 pound (454 g) bitter melon, sliced in half lengthwise and seeds scooped out

2 teaspoons (11 g) kosher salt

6 dried shiitake mushrooms

½ cup (120 ml) boiling water

2 tablespoons (30 ml) avocado oil, divided

1½ teaspoons (8 ml) toasted sesame oil

1 tablespoon (30 ml) soy sauce or tamari

2 whole organic large eggs, lightly beaten (optional)

2 tablespoons (30 ml) koregusu (Okinawan chili sauce) or sriracha (optional)

1. While the tofu is pressing, prepare the bitter melon.

2. Slice the melon halves into ¼-inch-thick half-moon slices and place in a medium bowl.

3. Add the salt to the melon, toss to coat, and allow to sit for 20 minutes.

4. Meanwhile, combine the shiitake mushrooms and boiling water. Allow to sit for 15 minutes. Reserve the liquid and save the mushrooms for another use (like the Miso Soup on page 120).

5. After 20 minutes, squeeze all excess liquid from the melon and transfer to a colander. Rinse with cold water and pat completely dry.

6. Once the tofu is pressed, cut into 1-inch (2.5-cm) pieces.

7. Heat a large nonstick sauté pan over medium-low heat. Add 1 tablespoon (15 ml) of the avocado oil and the sesame oil. Once hot, add the cubed tofu and allow to cook on one side for 5 minutes, or until lightly browned. Toss the pan and continue to cook another 5 minutes. Toss again, and cook another 5 minutes. Transfer to a bowl.

8. Heat the remaining 1 tablespoon (15 ml) avocado oil over high heat. And the bitter melon and cook, without touching, for 5 minutes. Stir and cook an additional 2 minutes.

9. Add the tofu back into the pan, along with the shiitake mushroom water and soy sauce. Cook for 1 minute, or until the liquid is almost evaporated.

10. If using the eggs, add them in now, scrambling.

11. Transfer the stir fry to a platter and drizzle with the koregusu or sriracha, if desired.

BITTER MELON AND TOFU STIR-FRY

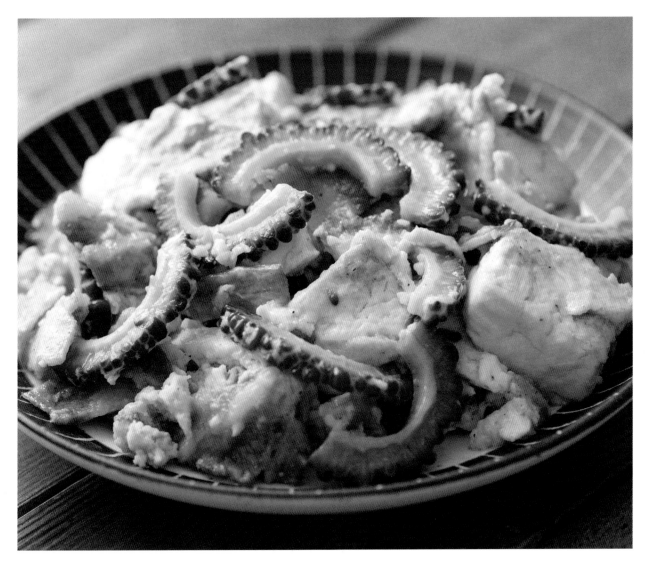

TENDER SEASONED KOMBU

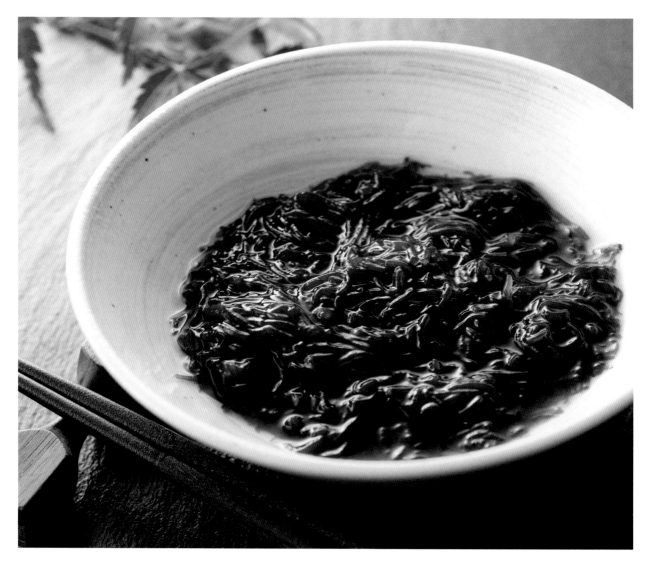

The type of kombu you use makes a huge difference in this dish! Try to find Hidaka kombu because it is tender and easy to cook. This dish also calls for bonito flakes, a unique form of smoked fish, traditionally skipjack tuna, that is smoked and shaved into flakes. Mirin is a type of rice wine similar to sake, but with a lower alcohol and higher sugar content. All three of these items can be found in an Asian market. Serve this wonderful dish as an accompaniment to steamed rice.

Serves 4

8 ounces (227 g) Hidaka kombu, simmered for 30 minutes

4 cups (946 ml) water

½ cup (120 ml) soy sauce or tamari

¼ cup (60 ml) sake

¼ cup (60 ml) mirin

4 teaspoons (20 ml) unseasoned rice vinegar

4 teaspoons (10 g) unprocessed sugar

1 teaspoon crushed red pepper flakes

2 teaspoons (6 g) white sesame seeds

2 teaspoons dried bonito flakes (optional)

1. Drain and cool the simmered kombu. (The broth can be saved to make homemade dashi; see page 119.) Cut the kombu into thin strips and transfer to a medium saucepan.

2. Add the water, soy sauce, sake, mirin, rice vinegar, sugar, and red pepper flakes. Bring to a boil over high heat. Reduce the heat to low and simmer, uncovered, for 20 to 25 minutes. The kombu should be really tender at this point, and the liquid should be almost all gone. If it's not tender, add a little more water and continue to cook for a few more minutes.

3. Remove from heat, sprinkle with the sesame seeds, and stir to distribute.

4. This keeps in the refrigerator in an airtight container for up to 2 weeks. When ready to serve, top with bonito flakes, if desired.

Kelp is the main way Okinawans take in essential minerals such as sodium, calcium, potassium, and iodine. This seaweed is the foundation of Japanese and Okinawan cuisine, and it adds an umami punch to dashi broth, which is the start to soups, stews, sauce for stir-fries, and so much more. Make a large batch and freeze for future uses. This dashi replaces the traditional bonito (fish) flakes with mushrooms. Try it either way!

Makes 8 cups

10 dried shiitake mushrooms

1 cup (235 ml) boiling water

9 cups (2.1 L) water

2 ounces (57 g) dried kombu (preferably Hidaka)

1. Soak the dried mushrooms in boiling water for 15 minutes. Drain and reserve mushrooms. (You can save the liquid for Bitter Melon and Tofu Stir-Fry on page 115.)

2. Add the fresh water to a large stock pot and bring to a boil.

3. Meanwhile, rinse the kombu under cold running water.

4. Reduce the heat to a simmer, add the kombu and mushrooms, and simmer for 20 to 25 minutes.

5. Remove from heat. Remove the kombu (use for the Tender Seasoned Kombu on page 116) and mushrooms, reserving the mushrooms for another use (like the Miso Soup on page 120).

6. Cool and store in an airtight container for up to 1 week or freeze for up to 6 months.

DASHI BROTH

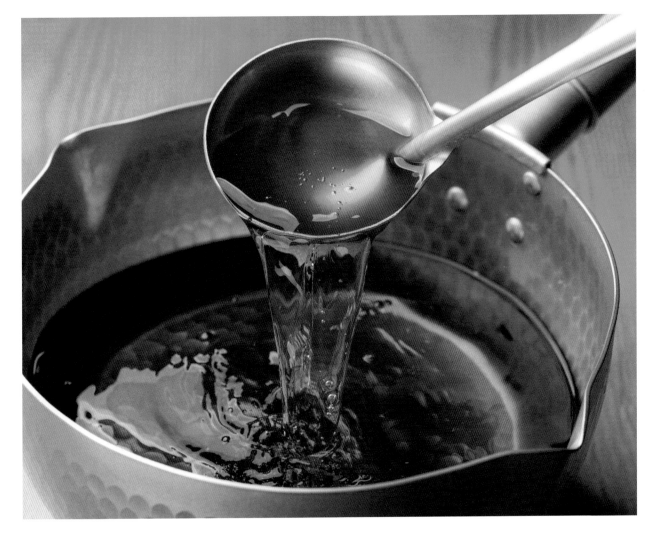

MISO SOUP

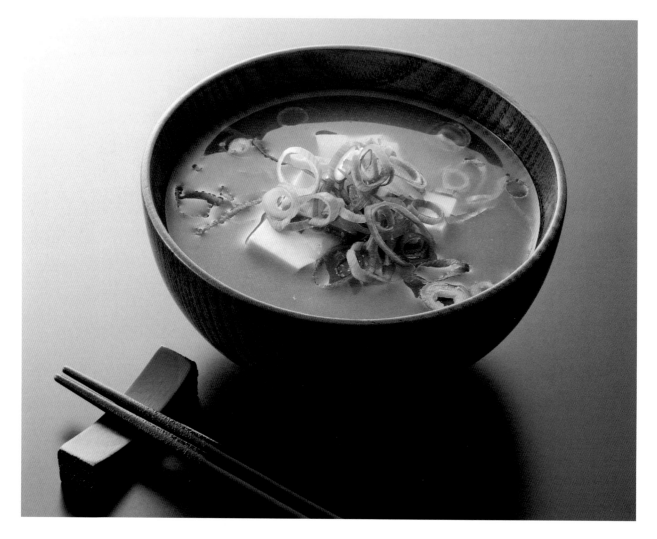

Okinawan miso soup is filling and nutritious—not a side dish. There are no rules to what you can and cannot put in your soup, just make sure to add lots of veggies. Eating miso soup is an almost daily occurrence in Okinawa; served at breakfast, lunch, and/or dinner, this fermented broth is so versatile. The vegetable-tofu version is much loved, but you will also find clam, pork belly, bonito flake, or even green tea versions; feel free to experiment and try them all!

Serves 2 large portions

4 cups (946 ml) Dashi Broth (page 119)

2½ tablespoons (45 g) white or other light miso paste

2 teaspoons (10 ml) sesame oil

1 carrot, peeled and thinly sliced on the diagonal (about ½ cup)

1 cup (84 g) bite-size pieces napa cabbage

1 cup (68 g) beech mushrooms or rehydrated dried shiitake mushrooms (use some from Dashi Broth or Bitter Melon and Tofu Stir-Fry, page 115)

6 ounces (170 g) extra-firm tofu, cut into ¼-inch cubes (about 1 cup)

¼ cup (16 g) thinly sliced scallions

Poached egg, crispy pork belly, bean sprouts, sliced onion (optional)

1. Bring the dashi broth to a boil over high heat. Remove from heat and whisk in the miso paste.

2. While the dashi is coming to a boil, add a little of the sesame oil to a sauté pan over medium heat. Sauté the carrots until crisp-tender, about 4 minutes. Repeat with the remaining sesame oil, the napa cabbage, and mushrooms.

3. After the vegetables are tender but still slightly crisp, transfer them to 2 serving bowls. Divide the tofu between the bowls.

4. Once the miso has dissolved in the broth, pour the soup over the vegetables and serve topped with sliced scallions.

5. Add optional poached egg, crispy pork belly, bean sprouts, or sliced onion to individual servings, if desired.

The sweet teriyaki–like sauce made with mirin, sugar, sake, and soy is a perfect combination to counteract the bitterness of the goya, or bitter melon. These little bites are perfect with a bowl of steamed rice and vegetables. You may substitute ground pork for the mushroom mince, if you prefer.

Serves 4

2 large (about ⅔ pound [303 g]) goya (bitter melons)

1 tablespoon (16 g) kosher salt

1 pound (454 g) fresh shiitake mushrooms, stems removed

4 tablespoons (40 g) potato starch, divided

2 tablespoons (30 ml) sesame oil

2 teaspoons (9 g) grated garlic

2 tablespoons (30 ml) sake

2 tablespoons (30 ml) soy sauce

2 tablespoons (30 ml) mirin

1 tablespoon (8 g) unprocessed sugar

1 tablespoon (15 ml) avocado oil

½ cup (120 ml) water

1. Slice each melon into 8 sections, for 16 pieces total. Remove the seeds and pulp with a spoon, leaving the circles intact. Place all in a bowl, cover with the salt, and stir. Allow to sit for 30 minutes. Drain, rinse well with water, and then pat completely dry.

2. Meanwhile, in the bowl of a food processor, add the shiitake mushrooms. Pulse off and on for 30 seconds to 1 minute, until the mixture resembles ground meat.

3. Transfer the minced mushrooms to a bowl and toss with 1 tablespoon (10 g) of the potato starch, the sesame oil, and grated garlic; set aside.

4. Now make the sauce. In a small bowl, whisk together the sake, soy sauce, mirin, and sugar.

5. Add the dried goya to a clean medium bowl and toss well with the remaining 3 tablespoons (30 g) potato starch, making sure the starch is coating the inside as well as the outside.

6. Divide the mushroom mixture between the goya rounds and set on a plate.

7. In a large sauté pan over medium heat, add the avocado oil. Once hot, add the goya and cook for 4 minutes on each side. They will be browned and crisp on both sides.

8. Add the water, cover the pan, and steam for 4 minutes longer. The water will be evaporated.

9. Reduce the heat to low, add the sauce, and cook for 1 to 2 minutes, or until the sauce becomes sticky and coats the goya.

10. Serve hot!

MUSHROOM MINCE–FILLED GOYA

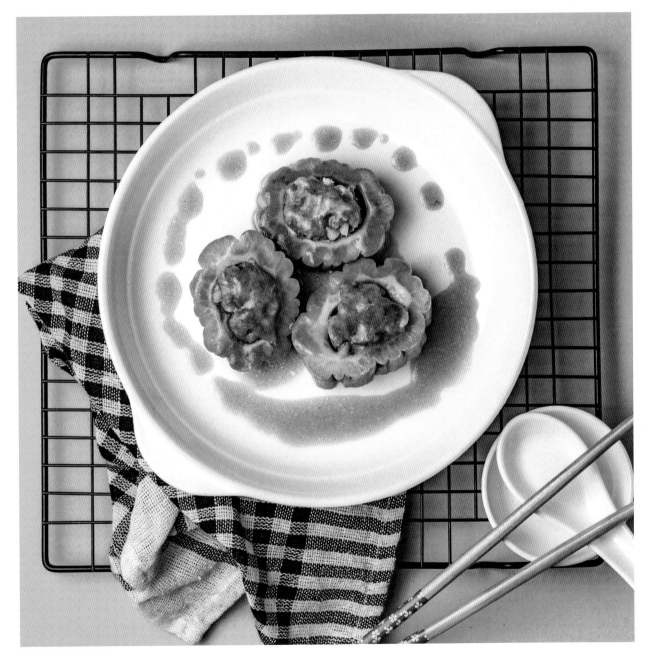

OKINAWAN MILK TEA

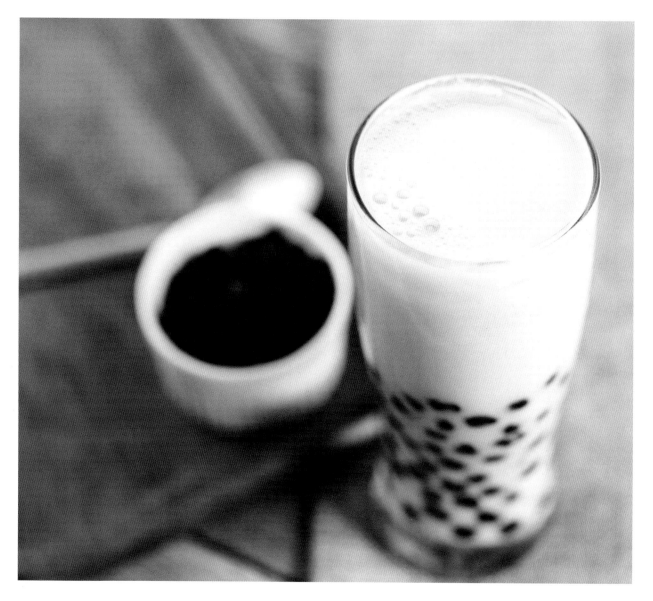

This tea is one of the healthiest types of bubble teas: black tea, kokuto sugar or Okinawa black/brown sugar, milk, and tapioca pearls. (These translucent spheres are made from the cassava root; large tapioca pearls can be found in an Asian market, but if you can't find them, opt for regular tapioca pearls that are easily found in your grocery store.) The tea is not too sweet because kokuto is a darker and healthier type of sugar made in Japan. It has a deep and rich flavor, made by squeezing sugar cane juice and boiling it down, making it higher in iron, calcium, and potassium.

Serves 4

½ cup (72 g) Okinawa black/brown sugar or kokuto

5¼ cups (1.25 L) water, divided

¾ cup (113 g) tapioca pearls

1 tablespoon (6 g) black loose-leaf tea (Darjeeling, Ceylon, Earl Grey, or Assam)

½ cup (120 ml) unsweetened oat milk creamer

1. To make the syrup, combine the sugar and ¼ cup (60 ml) water in a small saucepan over medium-high heat, stirring constantly until boiling.

2. Reduce the heat to medium-low and simmer until it's really thick, about 4 minutes. Watch carefully. Once thick, remove from heat.

3. In another small saucepan, bring 3 cups (700 ml) water to a boil over high heat. Add the tapioca pearls and cook for 6 minutes, or until they float to the surface. The time may differ depending on the type you get.

4. Drain the tapioca and add them into the sugar syrup. Turn the syrup on low heat and cook an additional 2 minutes. Remove from heat.

5. Boil the remaining 2 cups (470 ml) water in a saucepan or kettle. Turn it off and add the black tea. Cover and allow to steep for up to 5 minutes. Strain the tea leaves.

6. To serve, divide the tapioca pearls and syrup among 4 small heat-tolerant glasses. Top with the steeped tea, then the milk. Allow individuals to stir all together. For some extra decadence, top with a little extra frothed oat milk creamer!

These banana muffins have a rich, molasses-like flavor from the kokuto. They are delicious as a breakfast, snack, or dessert! Kokuto comes in rock form or in crushed form. If you can only find the rock form, you may process the rocks in a food processor to make it easier to use in this recipe.

Note: Kokuto (black/brown sugar) can contain the bacteria that causes infant botulism, so do not feed kokuto and these muffins to children younger than 12 months.

Makes 12

6 large ripe bananas

⅔ cup (95 g) kokuto sugar powder (not rocks), passed through a sieve

2 large eggs or equivalent egg substitute

½ cup (120 ml) melted coconut oil or butter

6 tablespoons (90 ml) water

2 cups (240 g) organic unbleached all-purpose flour, sifted

½ cup (48 g) almond flour

2 teaspoons (9 g) baking powder

½ teaspoon kosher salt

1 cup (128 g) pecan halves

⅔ cup (113 g) dark chocolate chunks or chips

1. Preheat the oven to 365°F (185°C, or gas mark 5). Line a 12-cup muffin pan with paper liners and set aside.

2. In a large bowl, mash the bananas with a fork.

3. Add in the kokuto sugar, eggs, coconut oil, and water. Mix until just combined.

4. In a medium bowl, mix the flours, baking powder, and salt.

5. Add the dry ingredients to the wet and mix until just combined.

6. Divide the batter among the 12 muffin cups and then top each one with the pecan halves and chocolate chunks.

7. Transfer to the oven and bake for 25 minutes, or until a toothpick comes out of the center one with little crumbs.

8. Cool for 5 minutes in the muffin pan, then remove and allow to cool completely on a wire rack. May be stored in an airtight container in the refrigerator for up to 1 week or frozen for 3 months.

KOKUTO, BANANA, AND DARK CHOCOLATE MUFFINS

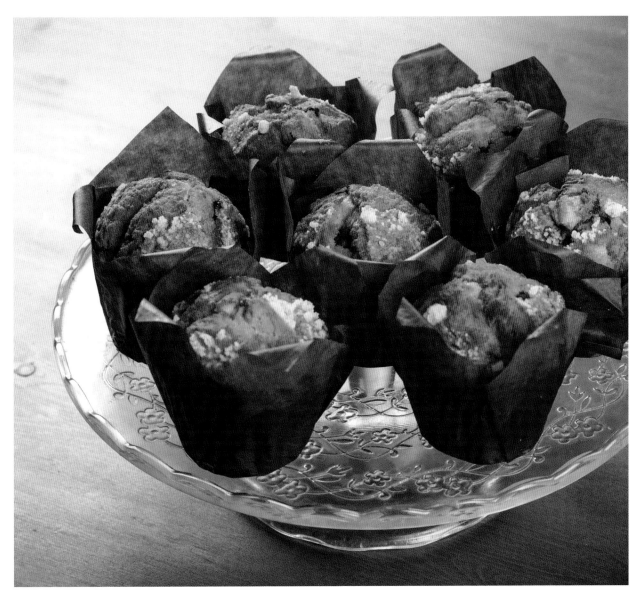

CHAPTER 6

SARDINIA, ITALY

This island off the western coast of Italy is a combination of mountains, forests, and beaches, small villages and larger cities, with a special blend of Italian culture and traditions, as well as incredible food and wine. As a Mediterranean island, it has an ideal climate with warm weather year round. Historical markers lie around every corner, reminding inhabitants of their rich traditions. Sardinia was first put on the world stage because of its large population of male centenarians. In fact, they have a custom for when people turn 100: they paint a scene of their life on the side of their home, which all the villagers can admire and celebrate.

A Day in the Life

In Sardinia, the bells of a local church ring every morning at 7 a.m., with the sounds of "Ave Maria," announcing that the day of praise has begun. The townspeople gather in the local cafes where copious amounts of coffee are served to wash away the laughter and wine of the previous night. Community is everything to this Italian island; starting and ending their days together, sitting around with family and friends is commonplace. Breakfast in Italy is not a very normal occurrence, and Sardinia is no exception, but coffee and a pastry such as a cornetto and a slice of hard sheep's-milk cheese is a normal start to the day.

By 9 a.m. all windows and doors are thrown open, allowing the fresh air to circulate and the community to get as much of it as possible before the heat of the day becomes unbearable. Tending crops and livestock, some fishing, and doing household chores is how the morning unfolds. Individuals in the community tend to hundreds of small gardens daily; small booths dot the main road, selling the fruits and vegetables that come directly from the farmers. Sardinians mainly eat a plant-based diet, leaving the little bit of meat they do eat for Sunday or special occasions. The small amount of dairy they consume comes from their grassfed goats and sheep.

Around noon, the windows and doors are closed, sealing in the little bit of cool air that is left from the morning. Fruits, vegetables, homemade whole-grain breads, and legumes create a lunch that is much needed after the hard work of the morning hours. When the heat is at its peak, the whole town takes a siesta, resting and recouping, from 1:30 to around 4 o'clock. Sometimes shops reopen after siesta, sometimes they don't: island life!

Most afternoons after siesta are spent with family and community. Elders are cared for in Sardinia, respected for all their knowledge, and are a huge part of daily familial life. Dinners are spent with community, drinking local wine, enjoying the fresh produce harvested that day, the fish just caught, and the breads and pastries just baked. Routine is paramount on this island, providing the comfort and tradition that Italy is known for, creating a slow daily life that consists of walking, communing, laughing, and enjoying one another. The only time routine seems to break is during one of the many religious or other types of celebration and feasts.

And just like that, the day comes to a close. Rising with the sun and settling down with the sunset are the way of life in Sardinia. Family is loved and respected from children to grandparents, hard work is thought of as a blessing, daily walks are taken up the steep mountainside beside the grazing sheep, meals with wine are enjoyed and even luxuriated over, and community is everything.

The Food of Sardinia

The food of Sardinia, divided into coastal and inland categories, is rich in history and hasn't changed much in its thousands of years. There are far too many ingredients native to Sardinia to feature in just one section, but I am highlighting some of those more-often used and showcasing the exquisite ways they are prepared. Like all the other longevity hotspots, the simplicity of cooking is made possible by what is available seasonally; the residents eat what the earth provides in the time she provides it. Meat and seafood play a role in Sardinian cuisine, but they take a side role when compared to the abundance of fruits, vegetables, beans, cheeses, and nuts (which make up about 90 percent of Sardinian sweets).

GOAT'S AND SHEEP'S MILK CHEESE The ideal climate of Sardinia gives way to perfect conditions for sheep and goats to graze. The types of cheese that are produced in Sardinia haven't changed, but the methods of how they are made have evolved and been enhanced with the times. The nutrients of these cheeses are more easily digested when compared to cow's milk. They are rich in selenium, zinc, calcium, and vitamin D, making them an excellent aid to the immune system and a promoter of healthy brain function.

CHICKPEAS Like all beans, the chickpea is rich in protein, making it a star of any recipe. This high-fiber bean is known for helping maintain a healthy weight by creating a feeling of satiety, helping to control blood sugar levels, and promoting heart health. It is also a good source of iron, magnesium, and potassium. The inclusion of beans in one's diet is shown to aid in a longer, healthier life.

EGGPLANT The culinary uses for eggplant are diverse, and its health benefits are equally as impressive: it is a great source of vitamins C, K, and B_6, thiamine, niacin, magnesium, phosphorus, copper, fiber, folic acid, potassium...and more! This powerhouse's fiber content, which is important for our gastrointestinal health, also helps our heart health by reducing the amount of cholesterol our body absorbs. It also contains manganese, an antioxidant that helps protect our organs from carcinogens. The natural color of eggplant is an antioxidant known as anthocyanin, which has been linked to stronger bones and reducing the risk of osteoporosis. Eggplant is also high in phytonutrients, which improve mental health by increasing the blood flow throughout the body and brain.

FREGOLA Fregola is a Sardinian pasta that looks like pearled couscous. It is made from hard durum wheat flour, rolled, sundried, and toasted to a golden brown. The resistant starch of fregola helps to maintain a healthy blood pressure and aids in digestion. Sardinians use this pasta in soups, stews, or just on its own with fresh vegetables and/or seafood.

BOTTARGA Bottarga is a staple in Sardinian cuisine, often called "golden caviar." It dates back to when refrigeration was nonexistent and salt was essential for preserving food. It utilizes an ancient technique of taking the egg sac of mullet (the most valued), tuna, or swordfish, salting it, pressing it, and then drying it for a few months. Bottarga comes in two main forms: in beeswax, which helps to conserve all of its healthy nutrients

and inhibits oxidation, or grated and sold in jars. This unique food is quite pricey, but a little goes a long way. Bottarga is packed with zinc, omega-3s, protein, calcium, vitamin A, vitamin D, and has been shown to be a natural cancer fighter.

FENNEL, GARLIC, AND ONION I hate to combine these gorgeous vegetables into one category, but they are often used together, creating a powerhouse of flavor—and health benefits. Fennel is used as a vegetable (the bulb), an herb (its willowy fronds), and a spice (the seeds). It is rich in fiber and vitamins A, B, and C. This natural diuretic also helps maintain blood pressure. Onions and garlic are part of the allium family, and the sulfur-containing compounds in them have been linked to a decreased risk of cancer, especially gastrointestinal cancer. Lowering cholesterol and blood pressure, and fighting inflammation are a few of their other superpowers. Onions and garlic also contain flavonoids and polyphenols, which are plant compounds with antioxidant properties that help ward off degenerative diseases.

ARTICHOKES This prickly thistle is a rockstar when it comes to health benefits. Containing vitamin C, vitamin A, iron, potassium, and other antioxidants, it's a whole food in and of itself. Artichokes also contain a lot of protein, offering more protein than many other vegetables at 3.5 grams per serving. These beauties contain fiber, which helps keep you feeling full while also lowering your risk for heart disease; they also contain inulin, which is a unique form of fiber that helps prevent gastrointestinal issues and enhances the absorption of minerals such as calcium. Artichokes are an immune-boosting food,

containing polyphenols, which help repair the cell damage that impairs our immune function. This veggie is also an excellent source of folate, which has been shown to be beneficial in reducing the inflammation that causes allergies and asthma, as well as promoting a healthy pregnancy. Last but not least, the artichoke contains flavonoids that help fight a number of specific cancers, especially pancreatic and breast cancers.

TOMATOES Just like tomatoes are a staple of Californian cuisine, they are utilized in so many ways in Sardinian cuisine. In addition to lycopene, tomatoes also contain substances called lutein and zeaxanthin. These carotenoids may help protect eyes from the dreaded blue light of digital devices; they also help ease headaches and eyestrain. Additionally, tomatoes are an excellent aid in reducing inflammation, boosting your immune system, and keeping your blood from clotting.

CITRUS These vitamin C bombs are an excellent way to strengthen the immune system and keep skin smooth and elastic. They contain B vitamins, potassium, phosphorus, magnesium, and copper. They are anti-inflammatory, cholesterol lowering, cancer protecting, and heart healthy. The flavonoids in citrus fruits may also help ward off neurodegenerative diseases such as Alzheimer's and Parkinson's.

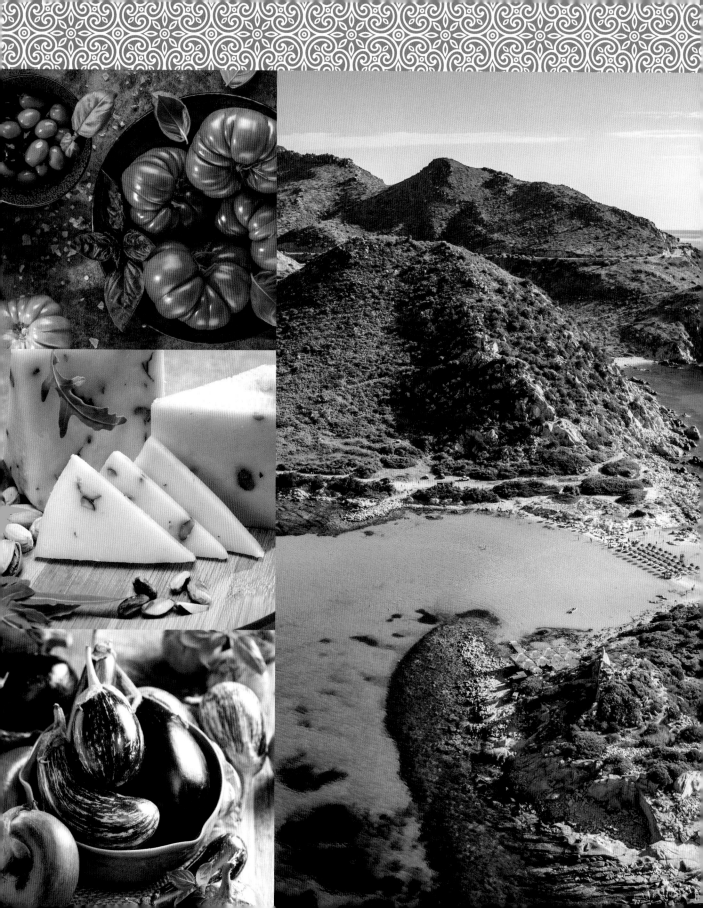

The Recipes of Sardinia

SEADAS (SARDINIAN CHEESE AND HONEY PASTRIES)

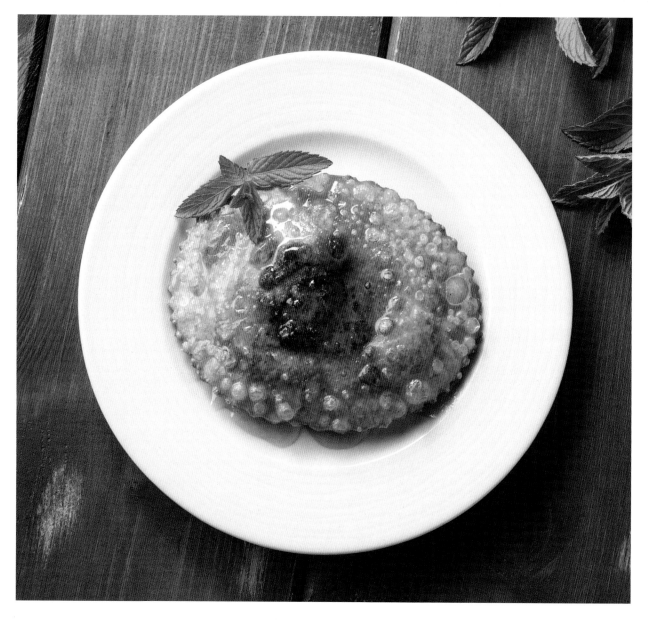

Breakfast is not very important in Sardinia or, for that matter, Italy. In fact, many Italians don't eat anything for breakfast, only needing coffee to make it through the morning. These pastries, which are probably the most traditional Sardinian ones, are light and crispy, filled with sheep's milk cheese, and drizzled with honey. Eaten on special occasions or just with a morning cup of coffee, these are delicious any time of day.

Makes 6

DOUGH:

2¾ cups (330 g) organic, unbleached all-purpose flour, divided

¼ teaspoon kosher salt

1 cup (235 ml) warm water (about 110˚F [43˚C])

FILLING:

2 cups (228 g) grated pecorino Dolce Sardo cheese or other mild fresh sheep's milk cheese

1 teaspoon lemon zest

FOR FRYING:

2 cups (470 ml) grapeseed oil

TOPPING:

½ cup (170 g) Sardinian or other good-quality honey

1. To prepare the dough: Add 2½ cups (300 g) flour to a large bowl. Stir in the salt to disperse.

2. Gradually add the warm water to the flour and knead until it comes together.

3. Sprinkle the remaining ¼ cup (30 g) flour on a dry clean surface and turn the dough out onto it.

4. Knead until it forms a smooth dough, 3 to 5 minutes.

5. Let the dough rest while you make the filling.

6. To make the filling: In a medium bowl, mix the cheese and lemon zest. Set aside.

7. To make the seadas: Roll out the dough to 1/16-inch thickness. Cut the dough with a 6-inch (15-cm) round cookie cutter. You should get 12 rounds. Lay the rounds out on a clean surface.

8. Place 1½ tablespoons of the cheese mixture in the center of 6 dough rounds. Place a second dough round on top of the cheese-filled one. With your fingertips, apply light pressure to join the edges of the two discs. Repeat for the remaining seadas.

9. In a large frying pan over medium-high heat, add the grapeseed oil and heat until it reaches 165˚F (74˚C). Line a baking sheet with paper towel.

10. Add a pastry and cook for 1 minute, or until golden brown; flip and cook until golden brown on the second side, about 1 minute longer. Using a slotted spoon, remove and drain on the prepared baking sheet. Keep warm while you fry the remainder of the seadas.

11. Drizzle with the honey and serve immediately.

This rustic herb soup, *s'erbuzzu* (or *s'erbuzu*), is made of greens, white beans, and pasta—in this case, fregola. Similar to minestrone, it's unique to Gavoi, a small commune in the mountains of central Sardinia. The herbs in this soup are traditionally foraged from around the island and can number more than a dozen, depending on the season. You can play around with the herbs and include something bitter, something floral, something grassy. Be like the Sardinians, and top it with a sheep's-milk ricotta salata, instead of the pecorino, if you wish.

Serves 4

2 tablespoons (30 ml) olive oil

1 cup (12 g) flat-leaf parsley, stems separated and minced, leaves coarsely chopped

½ cup (60 ml) dry white wine

2 teaspoons (6 g) fennel seeds

½ teaspoon kosher salt

¼ teaspoon freshly ground black pepper

2 quarts (1.9 L) vegetable or chicken broth

¾ cup (113 g) fregola

1 can (15.5 ounces [439 g]) white beans, drained and rinsed

4 cloves garlic, minced

6 cups (4 ounces [86 g]) baby arugula leaves, coarsely chopped

½ cup (6 g) mixed fresh herbs (tarragon, basil, dill, fennel fronds), chopped

¼ cup (25 g) grated Pecorino Romano cheese (optional)

1. Heat the olive oil in a large soup pot over medium heat. Add the parsley stems, wine, fennel seeds, salt, and pepper.

2. Bring the mixture to a simmer over medium heat and cook for 2 to 3 minutes, or until the liquid has evaporated.

3. Pour in the broth and bring to a boil. Lower the heat to a simmer and add the fregola. Simmer for 10 minutes.

4. Add the beans, garlic, and parsley leaves. Simmer 10 minutes longer.

5. Remove the soup from the heat and stir in the arugula and herbs. Check the seasoning.

6. Serve with grated pecorino on top, if desired.

SARDINIAN HERB, BEAN, AND FENNEL SEED SOUP

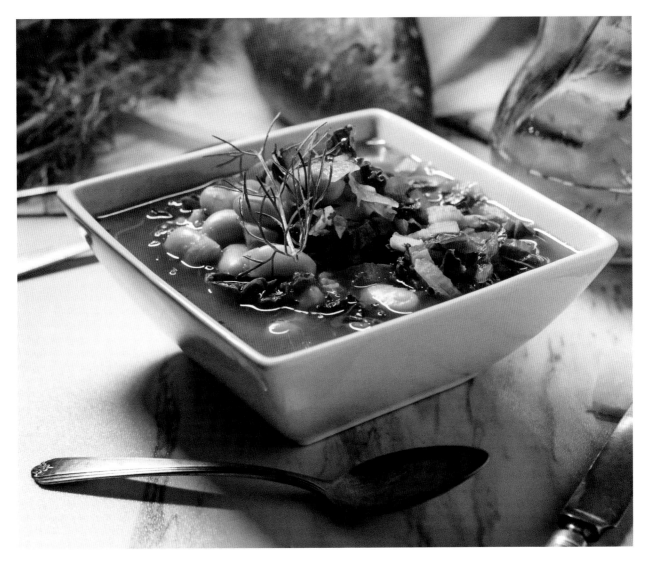

FREGOLA WITH WILD MUSHROOMS

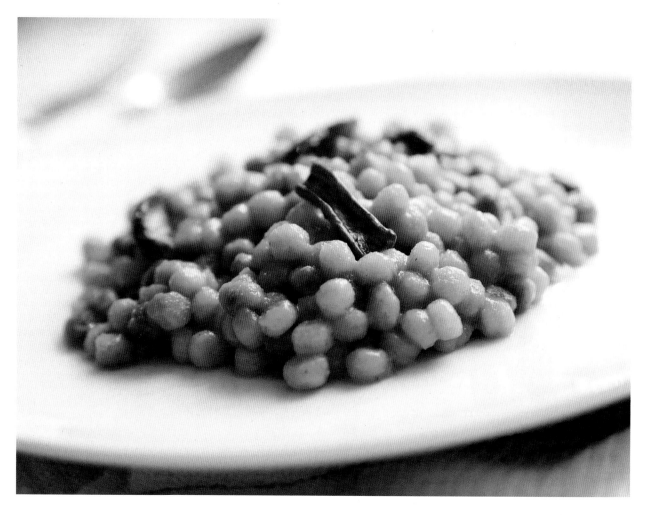

Sardinian fregola is a unique pasta with a toasted, nutty flavor that soaks up all the flavor that is added to it; it is easily found in specialty markets or online. This dish with wild mushrooms is elegant and satisfying enough to be the star of your meal—or it makes a perfect side dish.

Serves 4 as a main, 6 as a side

1 pound (454 g) fregola

1 tablespoon (16 g), plus ½ teaspoon kosher salt, divided

¼ cup (60 ml) olive oil

1½ pounds (680 g) wild mushrooms (cremini, oyster, porcini), chopped (about 6 cups)

½ cup (57 g) minced shallot

4 cloves garlic, minced

½ cup (60 ml) dry white wine

¼ cup (30 ml) good-quality balsamic vinegar

2 tablespoons (2 g) fresh marjoram, chopped

¼ teaspoon freshly ground black pepper

1. Bring a large pot of water to a boil over high heat. Add the fregola and 1 tablespoon (16 g) of the salt.

2. Boil for 12 minutes, or until al dente. Drain, reserving 2 cups (470 ml) of the pasta cooking water.

3. Meanwhile, make the sauce. Heat a large sauté pan over medium heat. Add the olive oil, mushrooms, and shallot. Sauté for 7 to 10 minutes, stirring occasionally, until the mushrooms are caramelized and tender.

4. Stir in the garlic and cook 30 seconds, until fragrant.

5. Add in the white wine and balsamic vinegar and bring to a simmer. Simmer until the liquid has almost evaporated, 5 to 8 minutes. The vinegar flavor will cook off, leaving a sweetness behind.

6. Add 1 cup (235 ml) of the pasta cooking water and stir to incorporate.

7. Add in the fregola, increase the heat to medium-high and simmer so that the pasta absorbs the sauce, about 1 minute. Add more pasta liquid if the fregola is too dry; you want it to be creamy and slightly wet.

8. Stir in the marjoram, the remaining ½ teaspoon salt, and pepper. Serve hot.

This pasta comes together quickly, so make sure you have all ingredients ready to make the sauce. The extra-starchy pasta cooking liquid, made from cooking the pasta in less water, makes a creamy emulsified sauce. Look for bottarga in specialty markets or online; if you don't want to grate it yourself, look for the jarred variety. This is a very elegant dish that will steal the show; serve alongside a gorgeous salad.

Serves 4

2 ounces (57 g) mullet bottarga, whole or grated (jarred)

1 tablespoon (16 g) kosher salt

½ cup (120 ml) extra-virgin olive oil

2 cloves garlic, peeled and lightly crushed

¼ to ½ teaspoon crushed red pepper flakes

12 ounces (340 g) spaghetti or linguine

1 cup (12 g) flat-leaf parsley leaves, finely chopped

1 tablespoon (2 g) finely grated lemon zest

1 tablespoon (15 ml) fresh lemon juice

1. If using whole bottarga, use a sharp knife to gently score the bottarga lobe down its length to expose the membrane. Using your hands, peel away the membrane and discard. Using a fine-toothed grater or rasp, grate the bottarga and set aside in a small bowl.

2. Bring a large pot of 3 quarts (2.8 L) water and the salt to a boil over high heat.

3. Meanwhile, in a large sauté pan over medium heat, combine the oil and garlic. Cook, turning the cloves over once, about 5 minutes. Remove the garlic with a slotted spoon and save for another use.

4. Add the red pepper flakes and continue to cook, stirring constantly, until fragrant, about 30 seconds. Remove from heat and stir in the grated bottarga. (Cooking bottarga is a big no-no, so be sure to do this step off the heat!)

5. Add the pasta to the boiling water and stir frequently for the first 30 seconds to prevent sticking. Cook the pasta until it is al dente, checking 2 minutes prior to package cooking instructions. (You will finish cooking the pasta in the sauce.) Reserve 1 cup (235 ml) pasta cooking water before draining the pasta.

6. Add ½ cup (120 ml) pasta cooking water to the bottarga mixture. Stir to incorporate.

7. Add the pasta to the sauce and rapidly stir and toss pasta until the sauce is emulsified, evenly coats noodles, and pools around the edges of the skillet, 30 seconds to 1 minute. Add more pasta cooking water in ¼-cup (60 ml) increments, as needed to adjust consistency of sauce.

8. Add the parsley, lemon zest and juice, and stir to combine. Serve immediately.

SARDINIAN PASTA WITH BOTTARGA

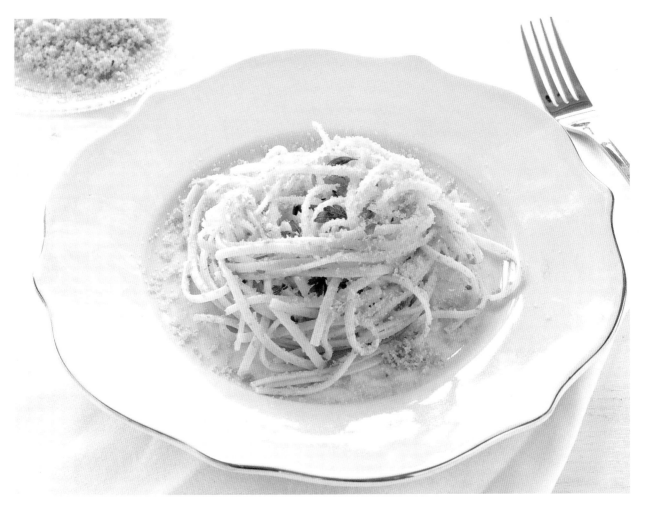

PANE CARASAU (SARDINIAN FLATBREAD)

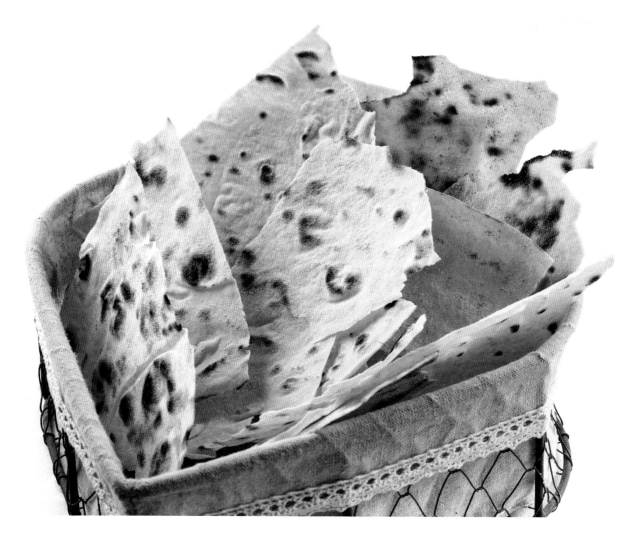

Pane carasau is a staple on the island of Sardinia, traditionally made for shepherds to carry for long stays in high pastures. Even though it's a yeast dough, it's a very thin bread—so thin, they say you can read sheet music through it. It is very versatile and can be served with any number of toppings such as olive oil; garlic and herbs; olive oil, garlic, and pecorino; or fresh tomato, garlic, and olive oil. It is best served for dipping into one of the Sardinian stews or soups (such as those on pages 137 and 150).

Makes 4

DOUGH:

1½ cups (350 ml) warm water (about 110°F [43°C])

1 teaspoon instant yeast

1 teaspoon sugar or honey

1½ cups (180 g) organic, unbleached all-purpose flour

1½ cups (245 g) semolina flour

1 teaspoon kosher salt

1 tablespoon (15 ml) extra-virgin olive oil

TOPPING:

¼ cup (60 ml) flavorful extra-virgin olive oil

½ to 1 tablespoon (4 to 8 g) coarse sea salt

1. In a large mixing bowl, combine the warm water, yeast, and sugar. Stir to combine.

2. Add in the flours, salt, and olive oil and mix to form a firm but soft dough, about 5 minutes.

3. Divide the dough into quarters.

4. Oil a large bowl, add the quarters of dough, cover with a damp towel, and allow to rest at room temperature for 2 hours.

5. Preheat the oven to 400°F (200°C, or gas mark 6). Line 4 baking sheets with parchment paper or silicone baking mats. If you only have one or two baking sheets, just repeat the process.

6. Using a rolling pin on a lightly floured surface, roll out each quarter of dough into paper thin rounds, about ⅛ inch thick.

7. Spread one of the thin dough rounds onto a prepared baking sheet and transfer to the oven.

8. Bake for 2 minutes. Remove from the oven, flip, and bake for another 2 to 3 minutes, or until the bread is crispy and lightly browned.

9. To serve, brush with excellent quality olive oil and sprinkle with coarse salt or any of the other topping ideas.

Fregola is a staple in Sardinia, used in soups, stews, or in recipes like this where it stands alone. Combined with saffron, tomatoes, and chickpeas, it comes together to make a complete and hearty meal. Saffron can be a pricey ingredient, but it's so worth it. The flavor is mild, sweet, floral, and has an earthy nuanced flavor. If you cannot find saffron or need a lower-cost ingredient, you can substitute turmeric for the color. This is considered a soup, but it's so thick, I think of it as more of a stew. Serve with some crusty bread (or Pane Carasau on page 142) for dipping.

Serves 4

½ cup (120 ml) dry white wine

½ teaspoon saffron threads

¼ cup (60 ml) extra-virgin olive oil

1 cup (142 g) finely chopped sweet onion

1 cup (170 g) cherry tomatoes, halved, divided

½ cup (71 g) finely chopped celery

1 tablespoon (14 g) minced garlic

½ to 1 teaspoon crushed red pepper flakes

10 ounces (283 g) fregola

1 can (15.5 ounces [439 g]) chickpeas, drained and rinsed

2 cups (488 g) strained tomatoes or tomato puree

1½ cups (350 ml) vegetable broth

½ teaspoon sea salt

¼ cup (3 g) fresh parsley, chopped

¼ cup (25 g) shaved pecorino Romano (optional)

1. In a small bowl, combine the white wine and saffron and allow to bloom for 5 minutes.

2. Heat a large heavy-bottomed stock pot over medium heat. Add the olive oil.

3. Once hot, add the onions, half of the cherry tomatoes, celery, garlic, and red pepper flakes. Sauté, stirring occasionally for 5 to 7 minutes, or until the vegetables are tender and the tomatoes are cooked down.

4. Add the fregola and chickpeas and stir to coat with the vegetable mixture.

5. Add the remaining cherry tomatoes, the strained tomatoes, vegetable broth, and white wine with saffron. Bring to a boil. Reduce heat to a simmer and cook for 15 to 20 minutes, stirring frequently, until the fregola is tender and the liquid is starchy.

6. Season with the salt.

7. Remove from the heat and sprinkle with the parsley.

8. Garnish with shaved pecorino, if you wish.

FREGOLA WITH SAFFRON, TOMATOES, AND CHICKPEAS

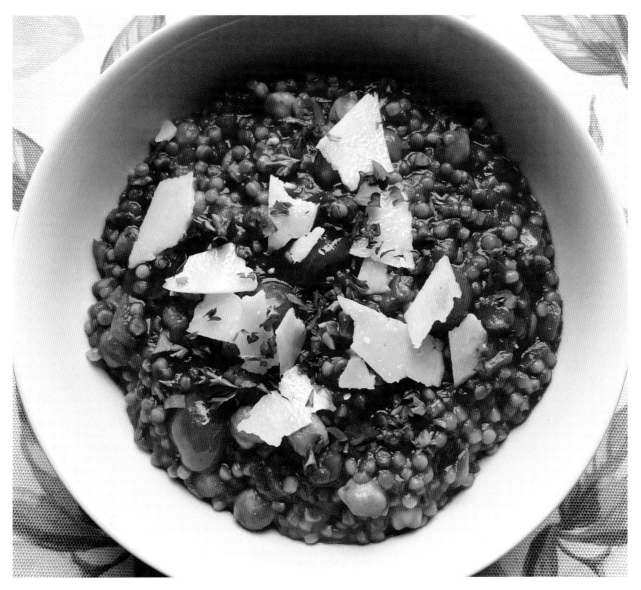

STUFFED AND ROASTED EGGPLANT

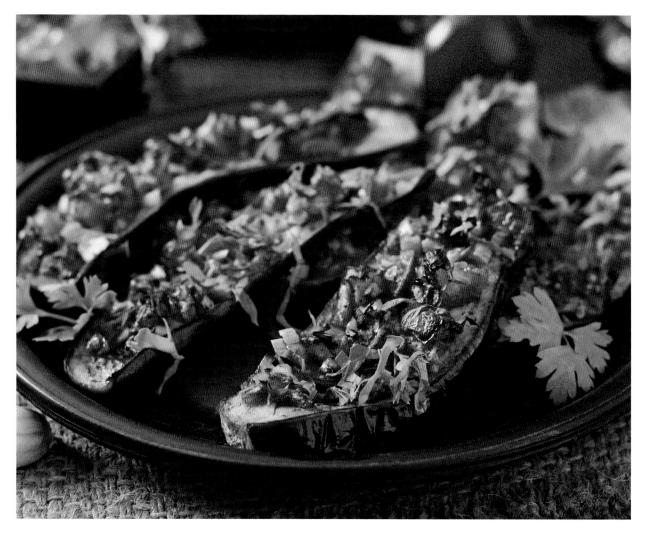

This simple dish is best when using in-season summer eggplants and cherry tomatoes for ultimate flavor and nutritional punch. Look for Italian eggplant with a firm, even-colored skin. They are a little different than American or Chinese eggplant; the shape is more globelike and less long. If you cannot find Italian, substitute American.

Serves 6

3 large Italian eggplant

¾ cup (180 ml) extra-virgin olive oil, divided

¼ cup (36 g) minced sweet onion

1 pound (454 g) cherry tomatoes, halved

1 jar (2 ounces [57 g] drained weight) capers, drained and rinsed

1 teaspoon minced garlic

¼ teaspoon crushed red pepper flakes

¾ cup (84 g) Italian seasoned bread crumbs, divided

¼ cup (63 g) tomato sauce

2 teaspoons chopped fresh oregano

2 teaspoons chopped fresh parsley

½ teaspoon sea salt

½ cup (50 g) grated pecorino Romano cheese (optional)

1. Preheat the oven to 400°F (200°C, or gas mark 6) and line a baking sheet with parchment paper. Set aside.

2. Wash and cut the eggplants in half lengthwise. Scoop out most of the pulp in each half, leaving ¼ inch of flesh on the inside of each shell. Set the pulp aside. Line a plate with paper towel.

3. In a large sauté pan over medium-high heat, add ¼ cup (60 ml) of the olive oil.

4. Once the oil is hot, add 3 eggplant shells and fry for 2 to 3 minutes on one side, flip, and cook another 2 to 3 minutes on the other side, or until lightly browned and tender but still able to hold its shape. Drain on the paper towel–lined plate. Repeat with another ¼ cup (60 ml) oil and the remaining eggplant shells.

5. Wipe out the pan, add the remaining ¼ cup (60 ml) olive oil, and set over medium heat.

6. Once the oil is hot, add the eggplant pulp and onion and sauté, stirring occasionally, for 3 to 4 minutes, or until tender and lightly caramelized.

7. Add the tomatoes, capers, garlic, and red pepper flakes. Cook, stirring occasionally, for 5 minutes longer, or until the tomatoes begin to break down and become a part of the sauce.

8. Remove from heat and stir in ½ cup (56 g) of the bread crumbs, the tomato sauce, oregano, parsley, and salt. Stir to combine.

9. Transfer the fried eggplant shells to the prepared baking sheet. Divide the filling among them and top with the remaining ¼ cup (28 g) bread crumbs and pecorino cheese, if using.

10. Transfer to the oven and bake for 20 minutes, or until they are lightly browned and bubbly.

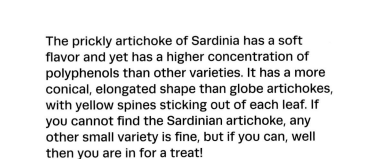

The prickly artichoke of Sardinia has a soft flavor and yet has a higher concentration of polyphenols than other varieties. It has a more conical, elongated shape than globe artichokes, with yellow spines sticking out of each leaf. If you cannot find the Sardinian artichoke, any other small variety is fine, but if you can, well then you are in for a treat!

Serves 4

1 lemon, halved

5 Sardinian artichokes or small baby artichokes

½ cup (114 g) ricotta cheese

½ cup (6 g) fresh parsley, chopped

1 tablespoon (15 ml) olive oil

1 teaspoon minced garlic

½ teaspoon sea salt

¼ teaspoon freshly ground black pepper

½ cup (50 g) Sardinian pecorino or pecorino Romano, grated

1. Bring a large pot of water to a boil over high heat. Squeeze the lemon into the water. Line a baking sheet with paper towel.

2. Remove any tough external leaves from each artichoke and peel the stem of outer tough skin.

3. Cut the artichokes in half and use a spoon to scoop the choke, or the furry thistle part, from the heart. Add the cleaned artichokes to the boiling water and continue until all are clean.

4. Boil all the artichoke halves for 5 minutes.

5. Remove all but two of the artichokes and drain on the prepared baking sheet.

6. Continue boiling the remaining 2 artichoke halves for 10 minutes longer, or until a knife inserted in the center comes out easily. Remove from the water and coarsely chop.

7. Add the chopped artichoke to the bowl of a food processor, along with the ricotta, parsley, olive oil, garlic, salt, and pepper. Blend until finely chopped and combined.

8. Divide the ricotta mixture among the artichoke halves and sprinkle with the pecorino cheese.

SARDINIAN ARTICHOKES WITH LEMON AND PECORINO

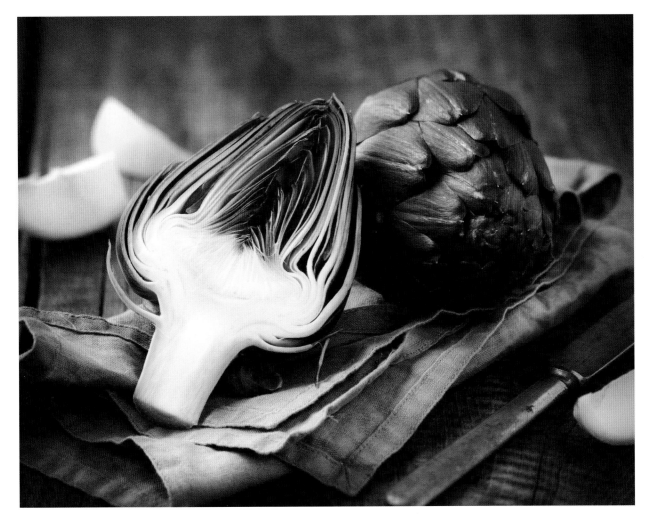

CHICKPEA AND FENNEL STEW

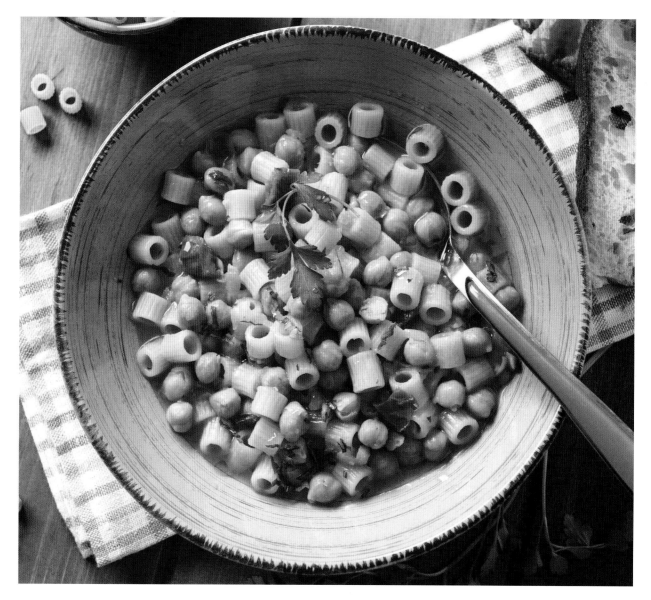

This hearty peasant stew is one designed to satisfy and nourish during long hard-working days. It is similar to the Northern Italian version of Pasta e Fagioli, but with ingredients native to Sardinia. Serve with Sardinian flatbread (page 142) for a wonderful and hearty meal.

Serves 4 to 6

1 cup (175 g) dried chickpeas, soaked overnight in cool water (8 to 12 hours)

2 bulbs fennel, stalks and fronds removed (½ cup [8 g] fronds reserved)

¼ cup (60 ml) extra-virgin olive oil

1 cup (142 g) chopped white onion

2 tablespoons (28 g) minced garlic

1 cup (134 g) peeled and diced russet potato

6 cups (1.4 L) vegetable stock

1 can (14.5 oz [411 g]) diced tomatoes, with their juice

¼ cup (38 g) ditalini

1 tablespoon (1 g) fresh rosemary, chopped

1 tablespoon (8 g) sea salt

½ teaspoon freshly ground black pepper

3 tablespoons (3 g) flat-leaf parsley, chopped

¼ cup (25 g) grated pecorino Romano cheese (optional)

1. Drain and rinse the chickpeas. Add to a large pot, cover with cold water, and bring to a boil over high heat. Reduce the heat to a simmer and cook until the chickpeas are tender, about 2 hours. Drain and set aside.

2. Meanwhile, halve, core, and thinly slice the fennel bulbs. You should have about 2 cups.

3. In a large stock pot over medium heat, add the olive oil, onions, and garlic and sauté for 7 to 10 minutes, or until lightly browned and tender.

4. Add in the sliced fennel, fennel fronds, and potatoes. Sauté for 7 to 10 minutes longer, stirring occasionally, or until the vegetables are tender.

5. Add the stock, tomatoes, chickpeas, ditalini, rosemary, salt, and pepper. Bring to a boil over medium-high heat, reduce the heat to a simmer, cover, and cook for 10 to 15 minutes, or until the vegetables are tender and the pasta is cooked through.

6. Remove from heat, and stir in the parsley.

7. Ladle into bowls and top with pecorino, if desired.

This simple three-ingredient dessert is delicious. Made with just orange peel, honey, and toasted almonds, they are entirely dependent on the best of ingredients. Using organic oranges is also a must! A great-quality, raw honey is also the star of this dessert, so don't skimp on that either. These beautiful cookies are traditional for ceremonies such as weddings and baptisms; originated in 1885 by the famous Nuoro pastry chef Battista Guiso, they are a showstopper. Although they are simple in ingredients, they do take a full day to make, so plan ahead.

> *Note: There are many tools to remove the peel from an orange; however, the old tradition of hand peeling with a vegetable peeler is best for this recipe. You want to make sure there is no pith or white part left on the peel, or you will have a bitter end result.*

Makes 24

3 cups (288 g) organic, thinly sliced orange peel (from 16 to 18 oranges, see Note)

3 cups (1 kg) raw organic honey

3 cups (342 g) slivered almonds

1. Place the orange peel into a bowl of cold water and soak for 8 to 12 hours.

2. After the orange peel has soaked, drain and dry on paper towels.

3. In a medium saucepan over medium-low heat, add the honey. Once warm, but not boiling, add the orange peel and leave it to cook over low heat for 30 minutes. The mixture will become thick and fragrant.

4. Meanwhile, in a small sauté pan over low heat, add the almonds and toast for 3 to 4 minutes. Make sure you watch them so that they are just lightly browned. Remove from heat and place in a bowl to cool.

5. Line 24 cups of a mini muffin pan with liners. Set aside.

6. Remove the honey mixture from the heat and stir in the almonds until coated.

7. Place 1 tablespoon drops into the mini-muffin liners and allow to cool slightly before serving. Store any left over in an airtight container in the fridge.

ARANZADAS (ALMOND AND ORANGE COOKIES)

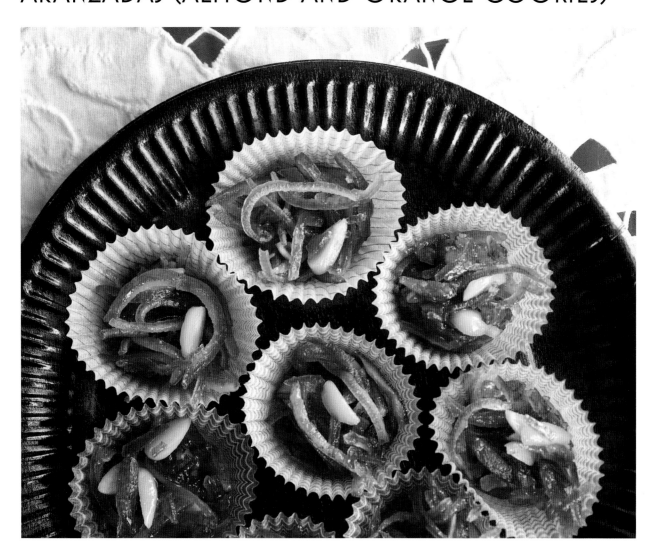

Bibliography

1. "5 Secrets for a Long and Happy Life, from Costa Rica's Blue Zone in Nicoya." Asuaire Travel Blog, 13 May 2020, https://asuaire.com/blog/en/costa-rica-en/5-secrets-for-long-and-happy-life-from-costa-ricas-blue-zone-in-nicoya.

2. @GCT, Greek City Times. "Why Ikarian Honey Could Be the Key to Longevity." Greek City Times, 19 Nov. 2019, https://greekcitytimes.com/2019/11/19/why-ikarian-honey-could-be-the-key-to-longevity/.

3. @ThePretentiousChef, Andy Anderson. "Italian Essentials: Sardinian Pane Carasau." Just A Pinch Recipes, https://www.justapinch.com/recipes/bread/flatbread/italian-essentials-sardinian-pane-carasau.html.

4. Avventura, Jennifer. "Daily Life." My Sardinian Life, 28 Feb. 2022, https://mysardinianlife.com/category/sardinia-sardegna/daily-life/.

5. Blair, Will. "Health Benefits of Lentils." WebMD, 22 July 2021, https://www.webmd.com/food-recipes/benefits-lentils.

6. BodyTalkDaily. "How a 100 Year-Old Farmer Stays So Young | the Art of Living | Tonic." YouTube, 7 Mar. 2021, https://www.youtube.com/watch?v=zxemFU8NHK0.

7. BodyTalkDaily. "The People on This Greek Island Live over 100 Years | The Art of Living | Tonic." YouTube, 14 Mar. 2021, https://www.youtube.com/watch?v=GP4ouNyTd0I.

8. Contomichalos, Steph. "5 Simple Rules of the Ikarian Diet: How to Eat for Longevity." Nefeli Nine, 6 Sept. 2018, https://www.nefelinine.com/post/5-simple-rules-of-the-ikarian-diet-how-to-eat-for-longevity.

9. "Coyol Wine." Academia de Español Nicoya. 8 Feb. 2019. Retrieved November 10, 2022, https://spanishschoolsincostarica.com/coyol-wine/#.Y21SjILMKqC

10. "Day in the Life: Ushi Okushima." Owaves.com, 7 Apr. 2021, https://owaves.com/day-plan/day-life-ushi-okushima/.

11. Doron, Tzvi, DO. "Friends and longevity: The Science of Social Connection." Ro Health Guide. 8 Apr. 2020. Retrieved November 10, 2022, https://ro.co/health-guide/friends-and-longevity/

12. "Festivals & Events." Sardinian Places, https://www.sardinianplaces.co.uk/guide/festivals-and-events.

13. "Fiestas Civicas de Cobano Costa Rica, Nicoya Peninsula." Peninsula de Nicoya Travel and Vacaton Guide, 13 Dec. 2021, https://nicoyapeninsula.com/cobano/cobano-fiestas/.

14. Fitzsimons, Jo. "Sardinian Diet – What They Actually Eat in Sardinia." 27 Sept. 2022, https://indianajo.com/sardinian-food-where-and-what-to-eat-in-sardinia.html.

15. Flinn, Allie. "8 Free Wordle Alternatives to Tease Your Brain." Well+Good, 12 Mar. 2022, https://www.wellandgood.com/wordle-alternatives/.

16. Hackl, Cathy. "What Costa Rica's Blue Zone Can Teach Us about the Future of Well-Being and Longevity." Forbes, 12 Oct. 2022, https://www.forbes.com/sites/cathyhackl/2020/08/12/what-costa-ricas-blue-zone-can-teach-us-about-the-future-of-wellbeing--longevity/?sh=72bb22e452d8.

17. Haworth, Diane and Michael Varbaek. "What Lifestyle Sardinia People Live." A Longer Healthy Life, http://www.alongerhealthylife.com/longevity-village/sardinia-italy-longevity-hotspot/what-lifestyle-sardinia-people-live-longevity/.

18. Hirschfeld, Tom. "Best Pane Carasau Recipe – How to Make Sardinian Flatbread," food52, 15 Dec. 2010, https://food52.com/recipes/8334-pane-carasau.

19. "Ikarian Food—Healthy Diet." Ikaria Travel and Holiday Guide, http://www.island-ikaria.com/about-ikaria/Ikarian-Food-Diet.

20. "Ikarian People and Lifestyle." Ikaria Travel and Holiday Guide, http://www.island-ikaria.com/about-ikaria/Ikarian-People.

21. Kubala, Jillian, MS, RD. "15 Simple Ways to Relieve Stress." Healthline Media, 20 Jan. 2022, https://www.healthline.com/nutrition/16-ways-relieve-stress-anxiety.

22. Lewin, Jo. "Top 5 Health Benefits of Miso." BBC Good Food, 17 May 2022, https://www.bbcgoodfood.com/howto/guide/health-benefits-miso.

23. MacVean, Mary. "Why Loma Linda Residents Live Longer than the Rest of Us: They Treat the Body like a Temple." Los Angeles Times, 11 July 2015, https://www.latimes.com/health/la-he-blue-zone-loma-linda-20150711-story.html.

24. Mariano, Kristin. "Okinawans Reveal Five Secrets of Healthy Lifestyle and Longevity." Travel Daily, 2 June 2020, https://www.traveldailymedia.com/okinawans-reveal-five-secrets-of-healthy-lifestyle-and-longevity/.

25. Mischke, Chiara. "Okinawa – Top 20 Must-Try Local Foods." Matcha - Japan Travel Web Magazine. 1 Aug. 2018, https://matcha-jp.com/en/6399.

26. Mleczko, Agata. "Daily Life in Sardinia." Null & Full, 26 Aug. 2015, https://blog.nullnfull.com/2015/08/26/daily-life-in-sardinia/.

27. NHSMyParea. "Get to Know the Cuisine of Ikaria." MyParea, A Family of Friends, 21 Dec. 2018, https://blog.myparea.com/cuisine-ikaria/.

28. Oliveira, Rosane, DVM, PhD. "Insights from Ikaria." Plant-Based Life Foundation (blog), 7 June 2017, https://pblife.org/health/insights-from-ikaria/.

29. Olive Oil Times. "People Here Use More Olive Oil than Anywhere Else in the World." Olive Oil Times, 11 Mar. 2022, https://www.oliveoiltimes.com/cooking-with-olive-oil/san-marino-leads-the-world-in-per-capita-olive-oil-consumption/97447.

30. Parker, Jenn. "This Country Holds the Secret to Living until 100." Culture Trip, 14 July 2017, https://theculturetrip.com/central-america/costa-rica/articles/the-blue-zone-diet-costa-ricas-secret-to-living-to-100/.

31. Pietracatella, Tania. "Sardegna's Secret to a Long Healthy Life." The Little Italian School, 7 Aug. 2020, https://www.thelittleitalianschool.com.au/blog/sardegnas-secret-to-a-long-healthy-life.

32. Pioli, Anna. "7 Essential Foods of Sardinia." La Cucina Italiana, 28 June 2022, https://www.lacucinaitaliana.com/italian-food/italian-dishes/essential-foods-of-sardinia?refresh_ce=.

33. "The Power and Nutritional Benefits of Seeds." 88 Acres, https://88acres.com/blogs/news/power-and-nutritional-benefits-of-seeds.

34. "The Prickly, Yet Tender Artichoke of Sardinia." Artecibo.com, https://www.artecibo.com/the-prickly-yet-tender-artichoke-of-sardinia.

35. Richeson, Lauren Paige. "How to Eat More Chan Seeds, a Dietary Staple in the Longevity Hotspot of Nicoya, Costa Rica." Well+Good, 22 Apr. 2022, https://www.wellandgood.com/chan-seeds/.

36. Robertson, Ruairi, PhD. "The Gut-Brain Connection: How It Works and the Role of Nutrition." Healthline Media, 20 Aug. 2020, https://www.healthline.com/nutrition/gut-brain-connection#TOC_TITLE_HDR_2.

37. Robertson, Ruairi, PhD. "Why People in 'Blue Zones' Live Longer than the Rest of the World." Healthline Media, 29 Aug. 2017, https://www.healthline.com/nutrition/blue-zones#TOC_TITLE_HDR_3.

38. "Sardinia Food and Wine." CharmingSardinia.com, https://www.charmingsardinia.com/sardinia/sardinian-food.html.

39. "Sardinian Cuisine, Identity and Flavour." SardegnaTurismo, 26 Jan. 2022, https://www.sardegnaturismo.it/en/sardinian-cuisine-identity-and-flavour.

40. Savor Japan. "Taste the Tropics! Okinawa's Specialty Dishes." Savor Japan, 4 June 2020, https://savorjapan.com/contents/discover-oishii-japan/taste-the-tropics-okinawa-s-specialty-dishes/.

41. Slobodian, Andrea. "Think Green! The Benefits of Fresh Herbs." Heinen's, 16 Apr. 2021, https://www.heinens.com/stories/the-benefits-of-fresh-herbs/.

42. Susanna Lobina. "Aranzada an Authentic Italian Cookie Made in Sardinia." Experience Sardinia.com, http://www.experiencesardinia.com/authentic-italian-cookie.html.

43. TasteAtlas. "8 Most Popular Sardinian Desserts." TasteAtlas, 13 Jan. 2021, https://www.tasteatlas.com/most-popular-desserts-in-sardinia.

44. Tavani, Claudia. "The Most Delicious Sardinian Food: Everything You Must Try." Strictly Sardinia, 8 July 2022, https://strictlysardinia.com/sardinian-food-guide/.

45. Toti, Daniela. "10 Healthy Foods from the 'Blue Zone' Sardinia." Hotel Gabbiano Azzurro Golfo Aranci, https://www.hotelgabbianoazzurro.com/en/Blog/10-Healthy-Foods-From-The-Blue-Zone-Sardinia.

46. Toti, Daniela. "Cheese of Sardinia." Hotel Gabbiano Azzurro Golfo Aranci, https://www.hotelgabbianoazzurro.com/en/Blog/Cheese-Of-Sardinia.

47. Vicenews. "The Tiny Island in Greece with the Oldest Life Expectancy in the World." YouTube, 14 Mar. 2021, https://www.youtube.com/watch?v=m2t2AWaRo1g.

48. Whiting, Kate. "Want to live a long, healthy life? 6 secrets from Japan's oldest people." World Economic Forum, 29 Sept. 2021, retrieved November 10, 2022, https://www.weforum.org/agenda/2021/09/japan-okinawa-secret-to-longevity-good-health/

49. Wooll, Maggie. "Start Finding Your Purpose and Unlock Your Best Life." BetterUp, 19 Oct. 2021, https://www.betterup.com/blog/finding-purpose.

Index